"The 1986 U.S. National Gymnastics Champion Jennifer Sey has a cautionary tale that every parent of an aspiring Olympian should read. . . . A candid, detailed, and often horrifying account. . . . Sey does not hold back in her honest analysis of the sport, coaches, parents (including her own), and especially herself. She comes across as an intense, sensitive, competitive, and endearing personality who makes her articulate and emotion-charged story accessible."

—*Courier Mail* (Queensland, Australia)

# CHALKED UP

## My Life
## in Elite
## Gymnastics

# JENNIFER SEY

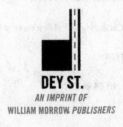

**DEY ST.**
*AN IMPRINT OF*
WILLIAM MORROW *PUBLISHERS*

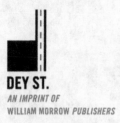

## DEY ST.
**AN IMPRINT OF**
**WILLIAM MORROW** *PUBLISHERS*

A hardcover edition of this book was published in 2008 by William Morrow, an imprint of HarperCollins Publishers.

FIRST HARPER PAPERBACK PUBLISHED 2009.

*Designed by Judith Stagnitto Abbate / Abbate Design*

Library of Congress Cataloging-in-Publication Data has been applied for.

ISBN 978-0-06-135147-1

HB 08.06.2020

FOR MY MOM

*United States Gymnastics National Champions 1975 to 2007,*
*as stated by USA Gymnastics, the governing body for*
*the sport of gymnastics*

| | |
|---|---|
| 2007 | SHAWN JOHNSON |
| 2006 | NASTIA LIUKIN |
| 2005 | NASTIA LIUKIN |
| 2004 | COURTNEY KUPETS AND CARLY PATTERSON |
| 2003 | COURTNEY KUPETS |
| 2002 | TASHA SCHWIKERT |
| 2001 | TASHA SCHWIKERT |
| 2000 | ELISE RAY |
| 1999 | KRISTEN MALONEY |
| 1998 | KRISTEN MALONEY |
| 1997 | VANESSA ATLER AND KRISTY POWELL |
| 1996 | SHANNON MILLER |
| 1995 | DOMINIQUE MOCEANU |
| 1994 | DOMINIQUE DAWES |
| 1993 | SHANNON MILLER |
| 1992 | KIM ZMESKAL |
| 1991 | KIM ZMESKAL |
| 1990 | KIM ZMESKAL |
| 1989 | BRANDY JOHNSON |
| 1988 | PHOEBE MILLS |
| 1987 | KRISTIE PHILLIPS |
| 1986 | JENNIFER SEY |
| 1985 | SABRINA MAR |
| 1984 | MARY LOU RETTON |
| 1983 | DIANNE DURHAM |
| 1982 | TRACEE TALAVERA |
| 1981 | TRACEE TALAVERA |
| 1980 | JULIANNE McNAMARA |
| 1979 | LESLIE PYFER |
| 1978 | KATHY JOHNSON |
| 1977 | DONNA TURNBOW |
| 1976 | DENISE CHESHIRE |
| 1975 | TAMMY MANVILLE |

# Foreword

"HELLO? HI."

"May I speak with Jennifer Sey?" An unfamiliar voice. Authoritative.

"This is Jennifer."

"Hi. This is Mike Jacki, the head of the U.S. Gymnastics—"

"I know who you are. Hi, Mike."

"I didn't think you'd remember me, Jennifer. It's been a long time."

"Over twenty years. But I remember."

"I'm calling because we need you. For an upcoming competition."

"I don't do gymnastics anymore."

"I know. But you'll have some time. A year. It has to be you. You're the only one with the grace. The poise. It has to be you."

I hem and haw a bit, forcing him to beg me to come back. Eventually I concede. I have to find a gym in San Francisco. I have to lose weight. A lot of weight, about forty pounds. I have to overcome my fear of climbing back onto the balance beam and the uneven bars. I'm thirty-eight years old. Is this possible? I want it to be, so I try. But I can't even perform the simplest moves. A handstand on bars sends me crashing. My weakened arms cause my hand to slip under my womanly weight. I land in a heap beneath the high bar, face bloodied from smashing into the fiberglass rail on the way down. My feet, bigger and wider than twenty years ago from giving birth to my two children, don't fit nicely side by side on the beam anymore. It used to feel as easy as walking on the floor, now it sways beneath me like a tightrope, my flat, heavy foot slips with just a simple step and I straddle the beam, coming down hard on my crotch.

I can't do this. I'll have to call and tell them no.

I'm such a disappointment.

And then, in a panic, I wake up. I ready myself for a day of work, troubled but wistful for a simpler time.

For years I have wrestled with my young life spent as a gymnast. When the present seems particularly stressful or uncertain, I dream this dream of being called back to the sport. I am so special, so memorable, so unique, that the Gymnastics Federation official needs me and only me. When, in my adult life, have I been deemed so exceptional that I am the only possible person who can fulfill a particular slot? Other than being a mom. And really, even the worst mothers are irreplaceable in the eyes of their children. So that confers nothing special. I must do it, I tell myself in my dream. I will train by myself. I will prove that this time I can do it on my own without the reproachful glare and abusive tirades of a coach guiding my every move.

The point of this dream is not lost on me. When life's options are either unappealing or unclear, gymnastics still seems the obvious and compelling choice. It harkens back to a time when all decisions were uncomplicated. I did it because it's what I did. Easy. The road ahead was well lit and safe. If I persevered, simply followed directions, I'd stay on course. I'd succeed. And if I didn't, I would not be to blame. It would be the faulty directions that caused my failure.

In my dream, I am reminded of all that was destructive and unhappy about my time toward the end of my career, the physical pain, the woozy light-headedness and hunger, the emotional desperation at having lost the only thing I had ever known. And yet, I also feel anxious because I can't go back. It's an impossibility. I wake in a panic. I must find my way now, as an adult, without anyone telling me exactly what to do.

This story—my story—is not intended to be an indictment of the sport of gymnastics. I was born with a competitive ire and near-manic ambition. Often this predisposition provides an edge in a highly competitive culture. At times, it morphs into self-destructiveness.

Gymnastics was the first excuse for me to turn on myself. I have repeated this behavior throughout my life. In college, my 3.8 grade-point average wasn't good enough; at work, my year-end review didn't earn me a promotion, meaning I might not make vice president before I turn forty; at home, when my son cries, he sometimes wants Daddy instead of me. This self-criticism turns desperate and frenzied, causing a variety of physical discomforts: wrenching stomach knots, heartburn, constipation, insomnia, headaches, infected cuticles from picking until I draw blood.

This is who I am. I am in constant psychic motion trying to better myself, beat myself, win. If gymnastics hadn't found me at age six, I would have found another childhood outlet for these inclinations.

I tried to tell this story in other ways. I shared it in snippets, when pressed, with friends who didn't know me when gymnastics comprised my entire identity. During college, I'd have to explain the lost year between high school graduation and the start of my freshman year at Stanford.

"What were you doing?"

"I was training."

"For what?"

"The 1988 Olympics. Gymnastics."

"Did you make it?"

"No."

Upon graduation, with little work experience to boast of, the "additional" section at the bottom of my résumé listed "1986 U.S. National Gymnastics Champion." In job interviews, this inevitably invoked questions. A former college football player who believed dedicated athletes to be the hardest-working employees gave me my first job because of my gymnastics accomplishments. The interview lasted for two hours, and all we talked about were the parallels between life and athletics.

Plagued by the dreams and roused by the interest of near strangers in my story, I wrote a fictional screenplay. It lacked the veracity required for emotional impact. I made a short film. And still, the dreams came. So finally, I just wrote the whole thing down.

This is a story about the ups and downs of my life as an internationally competitive athlete; as a young girl growing up in a world where underage and underweight girls were looked upon as cultural icons; as a fierce competitor in a culture where second place means losing; as a onetime winner who wasn't going to win anymore.

I was a girl who competed as a gymnast. I had fun and then I didn't. I lost and then I won. And then I lost again. I starved and then I ate and I thought I'd never stop.

But I did.

# PART I

1986

I'M WAITING FOR THE JUDGE TO RAISE HER ARM AND NOD HER head, signaling to me that it's my turn. Her polyester royal-blue suit with the crest makes her appear pathetically regal, like a homeless woman who used to be a traffic cop, still wearing her uniform with faded pride. Glory days.

I whip my head around when the audience gasps. Hope Spivey has fallen from the balance beam. The unthinkable has happened. Opportunity. She was the only true challenger left, and now she's on the ground, no longer perched high on the beam. She stands on the blue chalky mat, both hands on the plank, surely wondering how in the hell she ended up there. Her face is set with determination, but she is fighting tears. Her mouth is tightly pursed to control the tremor, which, if allowed to erupt, I know only too well would lead to hysteria. Tears have not yet spilled, but they are there. They pool behind her eyes, wet with disappointment, kept at bay with the sharp prick of her teeth into her lower lip. She must finish, despite the impossibility of winning. Despite the shame of falling, she must climb back up and continue. But for the moment, she wonders how she ended up on the ground.

I return my attention to the uneven bars in front of me. Almost time to go. The judge, head bowed, finishes calculating the score for the girl before me. She adds up all the deductions. There are always deductions. The elusive 10 has been driven to near extinction since Nadia hoarded them in 1976. Judges require audacious levels of difficulty to even start a routine at a 10. I am starting this routine at a 9.9, a tenth taken away before I've even begun.

I fold my toes under, jamming them into the bright blue mat, cracking them. *Crunch.* Both feet. I run my tongue across the self-inflicted canker, smooth and hot, on the inside of my lip. I check the chalk on my hands. Make sure it's just the right consistency: smooth but pasty, sticky enough to last the duration of my bar routine. I don't wear handgrips like most of the girls. I prefer hands to bars. No leather separating me from the feel of the smooth fiberglass. I don't trust that the bar is still there if the sensation is dulled by a leather barrier. Because of this, the skin on my palms rips more frequently. Whole calluses are torn away from my hand, leaving red, bloody holes. I trim the jagged remaining skin with a razor blade beneath my desk during math class, drawing stares from the boy next to me. I have a rip now. I've sanded and smoothed it with a nail file and covered it with extra chalky paste to dull the heat and pain of friction.

I take a deep breath. Exhale. Calm my breathing. Slow. Slow down. This is it. She raises her hand. I salute, one arm raised high above my head, chin up. "Go, Jen!" I hear my mother's squeaky voice from the stands.

I know I've won. It's my last event. All the challengers have fallen. I will win this meet. I'm in first place. I've never been so certain of anything. My blood is throbbing, pouring, crashing through my veins. The way water falls, without constraint, with limitless power. With certitude.

My heart pounds but not with fear or speculation. This is not the usual preevent "This is it, this is everything I've worked for and it all comes down to right now and I'll never get another chance if I screw this up." Not the usual "Everyone will be so disappointed but no one more than me because I've given everything for this and I can't see anything else, can't see past it, there's only this in my life." This time, my blood races and it roots me, tethers me to my true self. Gives me clairvoyance. This is not nerves. It is the opposite. My chest pounds with knowing. With the absolute utter certainty of knowing. With the strength and power and confidence of knowing that I've won. Of knowing exactly who I am. Deep in my chest, I've never felt so certain of anything, so sure of my existence. I am the next champion. It means everything to me.

I will not miss. I will win.

I am the 1986 USA national gymnastics champion.

It's over.

# 1972—1979

# Chapter 1

I LEARNED TO TURN A CARTWHEEL WHEN I was three years old. We lived in a white stucco ranch house on an air force base in Turkey that was connected to the neighbors' by a carport. Stephanie Manning, a strawberry blond hippie-haired thirteen-year-old, lived next door. She babysat while my mom visited with the other wives on the base. She taught me to turn my body into a wheel, my arms and legs the spokes, in between our Fiat and her family's station wagon. I felt unfettered and invincible. Special. Other kids my age could barely run, and I was turning perfect cartwheels on the cement without ever suffering so much as a scraped knee.

We went to Turkey in the fall of 1972, during the waning days of the Vietnam War. My father was sent there on the Berry Plan, which required that after completing his residency, he serve two years as a physician in the service, thus avoiding combat. He requested a remote assignment that allowed him to take his family. He was appointed as the pediatrician in the infirmary on the air force base near Istanbul, tending to the children of the families stationed there.

We moved halfway around the world, an adventurous prospect for my mother, who had envisioned a more traditional life as an upper-middle-class doctor's wife. They'd been high school sweethearts, and she'd put him through medical school, drawing blood from rabbits' hearts in a biology lab. A comfortable suburban existence was the least she could expect. But she embarked on the adventure, seven months' pregnant with her second child. Upon arrival, we lived in a trailer until being assigned housing. I liked the trailer because everything was miniature, perfectly tailored for me.

In December, after we moved into our base housing, my mother was airlifted by helicopter to the nearest birthing hospital, in Ankara. When she came home just before my first white Christmas, she brought my brother, Christopher. We had no long-distance telephone service. The phones only allowed us to call the other houses on the base. My parents sent audiotapes back home to my grandmother in Atlantic City, New Jersey, laughing about how fat and ugly this new baby was. They also sent pictures of me. My grandmother wrote a letter back scolding my Jewish parents for illicitly naming my brother after Christ while praising her first grandchild as a Joey Heatherton look-alike. I didn't know who Joey Heatherton was, but I assumed she was pretty.

When the snow cleared in the spring, my single cartwheel turned cautiously on the asphalt between the automobiles transformed into endless rows down the steep hill in our backyard. I loved the feel of whirling so fast that I was on the brink of losing control. I'd lose my bearings, spinning from bodily memory and sheer gravity, landing in a heap at the bottom of the dell. I'd tear back up the hill and do it again, audacious and exhilarated. When I'd yell for my mom, she'd come to the back window and watch me spin myself into giggly, dizzy fits. But mostly she left me alone, free to play without parental interference. I'd pass whole afternoons turning down that hill, invigorated by pure speed and independence.

I'd return home at dusk, ready for dinner. I'd make my famous pretzel-and-cheese salad. Not very saladlike, this concoction consisted of torn-up yellow processed cheese and pretzel sticks. My parents indulged me and served this with our meal every night. They even pretended to eat it.

I was permitted to make many of my own decisions. And live with the consequences. My parents were committed to not overprotecting their children, to teaching us lessons by allowing us to make mistakes. They did this in small ways, not dangerous ones. When I chose to wear my red raincoat in twenty-below-zero weather, I was cold. When I refused to go to sleep until they did, I was tired and grumpy in preschool the next day and the teachers were short-tempered with me. When I said I wanted more broccoli with dinner—*all* the broccoli in the bowl on the table—I was forced to eat it all and became sick with an unbearable stomachache.

Heavily influenced by the popularity of Dr. Benjamin Spock and his book *The Common Sense Book of Baby and Child Care,* my parents were avid practitioners of his philosophy: treat your child as a person, an individual, rather than a thing to be trained and disciplined. By the time I was four, I was the embodiment of Spock-fashioned, parental-inspired spirited individualism.

In 1974 we returned to the States and bunked with my maternal grandmother in Atlantic City. Nannie, as we called her, was hesitant to take us in, compulsive about the cleanliness of her home and particular about the designation of knickknacks in her living room. She kept plastic runners on the lime-green carpet at all times to prevent wear-out. She covered her white vinyl couch with green piping (it matched the rug) with even more plastic to avoid stains on the stainproof fabric. She followed drink-wielding guests (her family in this case) around with a can of Pledge and a damp dishrag, wiping up tables to prevent glass rings.

When I demanded a fruit-adorned decorative plate for my postdinner cookies, my grandmother was flattered. I'd taken note of the carefully-thought-through details of her decorating scheme. Though the plate was perched high on a frieze adorning the kitchen's molding, she obliged me, pulling a stepladder from the laundry room to fetch the dish for her only granddaughter. At sixty, she was agile as she climbed the steps on her tiptoes in glamorous heeled house slippers. I was smug even as my mother urged me to let my grandmother off the hook, tell her I didn't really want the plate with purple plums on it. But I did want it. And I didn't see why she shouldn't go to any lengths to get me what I required. When Nannie pulled it triumphantly from the shelf, I smiled a self-satisfied smile and ate my cookies like the Joey Heatherton–like star of the family that I knew myself to be.

As I was integrating into life in the United States, television fascinated me. In Turkey, I entertained myself with tumbling in the backyard, helping my mom prepare the meals, and tormenting my baby brother. In Atlantic City, I sat in front of my grandmother's cabinet-style TV watching Merv Griffin and Dinah Shore interview the stars of the mid-seventies—the Osmonds, Diana Ross, Donna Summer. Each of these guests sang upon introduction, usually accompanied by the host. Then they'd sit down in a living room type of setup and casually discuss their latest career endeavors. I was most intrigued by their disco-era outfits, which were always nighttime sparkly, despite the afternoon time slots for these programs.

I watched with my uncle Bobby, my mom's younger brother.

Bobby was born with Down's syndrome in 1952, when my mom was ten and my aunt Jill was five. From that moment he became my grandmother's sole focus, her entire life. Growing up, the girls were afterthoughts in the house as all attention and concern were dedicated to Bobby. A normal childhood for my mom and her sister was out of the question. Friends were not permitted to come over; in the 1950s it was an embarrassment to have a disabled child. The girls were left to fend for themselves while my grandmother devoted her life to caring for a child that would stay a child forever.

After just a few short weeks at my grandmother's, she asked us to leave. The chaos that two small children created was just too much for her. She preferred things neat and quiet, and we made that impossible. Calm consistency was critical in maintaining Bobby's daily care. She needed to implement an unvarying routine for Bobby to avert temper tantrums, and I often got in the way of that. He reserved a worn spot on the carpet for sitting cross-legged and watching television just inches from the set. He liked to bang two mangled white combs together while he enjoyed his shows. If I occupied that spot, his spot, even when he wasn't about to plunk himself down for an afternoon of Merv Griffin, he threw a tantrum. He screamed and pounded himself in the head, sometimes even wet his pants. His despair was agonizing for my grandmother. It was time for us to go.

We moved into a modest ranch house in Cherry Hill, New Jersey. My dad did a short stint in endocrinology at Saint Christopher's Hospital for children in Philadelphia before starting up his own office in Northeast Philly. A burgeoning practice, hospital moonlighting, and an hourlong commute across the Delaware River each day kept him very busy. Though he wasn't home much, my mother was happy, finally settling into her role as a doctor's wife. She had her own home, a brand-new car—a white Camaro with red-leather interior and an eight-track tape player—and the good fortune to give her children all the attention and opportunity that she had been denied.

I was happy, too. Our ample front lawn provided plenty of room for turning cartwheels. And now that we had a television of our own, I was free to watch the shows I wanted. I often tuned in to *ABC's Wide World of Sports* on Saturday afternoons; Olga Korbut quickly became my hero. I loved all the Russian gymnasts—Nellie Kim, Ludmilla Tourischeva—but the Belarussan pixie who won three gold medals at the 1972 Olympics was my favorite. She not only dominated those Munich Games, she charmed the world with her daring originality, charismatic smile, and lopsided pigtails. She single-handedly popularized the sport, turning it over to the little girls of the 1970s. Prior to Korbut's reign, gymnastics had been dominated by grown women. Larissa Latynina, holder of eighteen Olympic medals, had even competed while pregnant in the late 1950s and returned to the sport after giving birth to a daughter.

Olga was fearless. She was the first to perform a no-handed back flip on the balance beam. She also threw herself through the air, originating the Korbut Flip, a graceful backward-flying somersault on the uneven bars, caught midair. It was the first release move ever performed by a female gymnast on bars. Documentary footage, shown before the televised competitions, detailed Korbut's 1973 tour of the United States. The pigtailed sprite in the white leotard with red trim around the neck, adorned with a CCCP patch at the V, had little girls lined up to see her all across the country. Despite cold war tensions, President Nixon greeted her at the White House; he was "impressed with her ability to always land on her feet." She was a cultural phenomenon.

All the little girls of the 1970s wanted to be Olga Korbut. Until Nadia Comaneci came along with her fourteen-year-old, Romanian, 10.0 perfection. She was younger, cuter, and even more courageous than Olga. Her leotard with the yellow-and-red stripes down the sides appeared unthinkably technical and modern. She was the future. Her back arched effortlessly, her toes pointed beyond what seemed possible, her ponytail was uncommonly smooth, and her dark hair ultra-shiny.

In 1976 I was glued to the TV set for the Montreal Olympics. Nadia was the first gymnast to score a perfect 10.0 in the Games. It had been done before but never during the Olympics. She was perfect. Seven times over, she was perfect. Olga competed that year also, winning only a single team gold this time. No individual medals, Olga was already over the hill. The commentators shook their heads sadly as they announced Olga past her prime. What she had started four years earlier—making gymnastics a sport for young girls—Nadia continued in '76. Comaneci was only fourteen when she dominated, winning the all-around (the total scores of all the events), uneven bars, and balance beam. I watched Nadia with all the other little girls across the nation, convinced that this little girl's game was one I wanted to be a part of. I was seven years old already. I needed to hurry up and get going if fourteen was the magic age that brought champions to life.

I was already enrolled in hourlong weekly classes at The Gymnastics Academy in Cherry Hill, a local gym with an appropriately official-sounding name for parents interested in herding their girls toward Olympic stardom. My Nadia discovery prompted increased intensity. I demanded a three-day-a-week class schedule and my mother obeyed, submitting to the attending fees and chauffeuring requirements.

All of the parents, like the girls, were enamored of Olga and Nadia as well as the American darling, Cathy Rigby.

Though Rigby hadn't collected the piles of 10.0s and medals that her Russian and Romanian counterparts had, she was the first American gymnast to medal in world competition. Posters of her adorned the walls of the academy. In one she smiled, legs splayed in a perfect 180-degree straddle position on the beam, blond pigtails crooked and adorned with white yarn ribbons; in another, she was accepting the silver balance beam medal at the 1970 World Championships. She was homegrown proof that democracy and capitalism could produce world-class athletes. And her post-gymnastics success in show business, playing Peter Pan on Broadway, was all the more evidence that America was better than Communist Eastern Europe.

Having studied the myriad television specials and *Wide World of Sports* segments dedicated to Nadia, I decided I also needed to take ballet classes. Dance was a critical part of Nadia's schooling at the training center in Onesti, Romania, as grace was considered a requirement in the balance beam and floor exercise. While the girls in Russia and Romania were shipped off to factorylike sports academies, their families' well-being provided for if they succeeded in bringing glory to their countries with international medals, I signed up for gymnastics and ballet in the name of recreation. For the most part.

Of course I had fanciful dreams of glory, but there was no substance behind those idealized notions. I had no real understanding of the work, sweat, and sacrifice that would need to go into something like that. Neither did my parents. Of course, they thought I was special, as all parents think their kids are. But special in a contained kind of way. Maybe I'd make the high school gymnastics team, compete in state competitions, learn a little something about hard work and sacrifice. But all within reason. Nadia was enchanting, but Olympic medals were a dream for other people, for Eastern Europeans who needed a champion to ensure that their families had food on the dinner table.

My parents signed me up for gymnastics and supplemental ballet classes, hoping I'd have a little fun, get some exercise, get out of the house for a few hours. Pigtails and tutus, leotards and pincurls. It began with such innocent promise. How could anything bad come of this?

By the first grade, I was caught up in the frenzy of opportunity that is afforded to American youth of middle class standing. At the same time, I developed an accompanying sense of inadequacy. It began with a single art class right after we returned to the States. My mom signed me up for my first activity at the Jewish community center when we first moved to Cherry Hill. It wasn't that I'd shown any particular aptitude or liking for art. But it was something to do. All I know is that when we were supposed to draw a dog on that very first Saturday morning, mine appeared disjointed, flat, undimensional. Practically deformed compared with the elaborate depictions the other children in the class whipped up. The teacher hovered over my shoulder. "Huh," she said before moving on to the next child. Strike that one off the list. Art was not going to be my thing. The next Saturday, I cried, pleading with my mom to let me off the hook. It was such a small thing, but the lack of praise from the teacher had shamed me. I never went back to class.

Later, on a visit to Washington, D.C., as I walked with my dad to the Lincoln Memorial, I confidently informed him that I was quite good at math. First-grade addition and subtraction came easily to me. Perhaps I should consider a future in mathematics, I pondered aloud. "Girls aren't good at math," my father asserted. "Girls are better in the language arts." My dad was not a backward-thinking antifeminist. As a doctor, he believed what he said to be scientific and factual. But, again, this lack of praise disheartened me. The absence of encouragement felt like ridicule.

Then there was my greatest weakness. Music. Singing. I couldn't (and still can't) carry a tune. I couldn't hit a note. But how I enjoyed belting out Simon and Garfunkel's "Cecilia," one of my favorite songs from my parents' record collection. One summer day, while practicing cartwheels on the sprawling Cherry Hill front lawn, I sang: *"you're breakin' my heart, you're shakin' my confidence daily."* Amidst the cacophony of my own voice, I heard my aunt Jill say, "God, Merle, can you hear that? She can't sing a note. It's horrendous." My mom laughed. Then Aunt Jill turned to me. "I wouldn't take up music if I were you."

Why was everyone so anxious to tell me that I sucked?

When I stood out in gymnastics classes and was instantly acknowledged by the teacher as the "best one," I was joyous. Each time I was called upon to demonstrate handstand forward rolls, back walkovers, and back bends for the other kids, I was elated. And ballet was no different. Physical activity that required precision and technique was my forte. My ballet teacher often asked me to exhibit my pliés and my jetés. I did so with a smug grin, pleased with myself but aware that I shouldn't gloat too much, lest I make the other girls feel bad about themselves and resent me. And that would defeat the purpose of being good at something—to make people like me. To be admired. I just wanted everyone to be impressed. Being me was not going to be enough. I knew that. I had to exhibit some special skill to invoke this kind of affection.

I heaved a great sigh of relief. Finally, I thought, something I'm good at. One year back in the States, barely through my first year of elementary school, and I was already impatiently desperate to be the best at something.

**Chapter 2**  IN THE FALL OF 1976, AFTER A SUMmer of bicentennial celebrations in Philadelphia and obsessive Olympic watching on our side of the river in New Jersey, I attended second grade at the Haddonfield Friends School. This private Quaker school was one suburban town over from our less affluent starter-home neighborhood. Though we couldn't yet afford a house in Haddonfield, my dad scraped together the money to send me to school there. Both of my parents were intent on giving me the opportunities that they felt they'd been denied, having been raised by parents of modest means and frugal mind-sets.

My parents considered me to be smart, special in many ways. It was important to them that I receive the right education in addition to experiencing all of the extracurriculars so that I could become "something." I intuited that something exceptional was the hope, if not the expectation. It instilled a sense of always needing to strive for something more, better, "out there." I wondered: Could a thing—whatever it was—really be worth having if it was well within my reach?

Three days a week I'd go from pink-tights/black-leotard ballet class with Miss Claire to gymnastics practice with Rich and Debbie Tobin, spiffy in my bright orange "leo." In the front seat of the car, I wiggled out of my boring ballet uniform, inhaling a Milky Way to hold me over until dinner. My brother, Chris, almost three years my junior, sat quietly in the backseat, trailing obediently from one location to the next. Where I went, he went.

On Saturdays, when there was no ballet class first, my mom and I had violent screaming matches before gymnastics practice. She could never pull my hair tightly enough, perfectly back into a ponytail without "bumps." Heather's hair never had bumps. She was only one year older than me and already in the enviable position of being on the Cabrielles, the competition team at The Gymnastics Academy. I was convinced the imperfect bumps in my hair were holding me back. I panicked about whether I would make the team, like Heather, before I turned eight. How would I be able to enter competitions, get my perfect 10, if my mom couldn't even do my hair right. The anger would seethe in me, flushing my cheeks, bringing hot tears and vicious screams. It was frightful. I was a mere child, but I howled with rage at the utter unacceptability of my mom's ponytail-making skills. But she scrambled, trying to make my hair perfect. She bought a vast array of brushes, praying they'd make my hair smoother. She'd brush the hair back over and over and again, applying more and more hair spray. Yet she was always met with disapproval. Nothing was good enough for me.

Heather's hair was always glossy and smooth. Her widow's peak allowed for a flawless sweep into a highly perched pigtail. Blond and perky, she was Cathy Rigby's obvious successor. She had natural muscles in her legs, a defined quadriceps above her knee, indentations beside the tendons that ran over her hips. She seemed to be blessed with Nadia's body and Cathy's Rigby's sun-kissed appearance.

I, on the other hand, was not blond. Or tan. I felt chubby and awkward, even then. There were no sinewy muscles announcing themselves on my thighs. I looked for them in vain, tried to create them with extra wall sits after class and long rides on my purple banana-seat bicycle. I was serious and competitive, even then. I wanted to become Heather's teammate and friend, but I also wanted to be better than she was. I wanted the coaches to acknowledge me as the one who did the straightest handstands and the highest back flips.

When I stayed to watch the team girls after my class ended, I saw Heather flying through the air, performing layouts (straight-bodied, no-handed back flips) on floor. I was still mastering back handsprings and attempting back tucks (handless somersaults with the body folded into a ball). My fear of injury got in the way of conquering the more difficult skills as quickly as some of the other girls in my class. According to Rich, the head coach and gym's owner, apprehensiveness was preventing me from moving up to the Cabrielles. It wasn't my hair, as I'd suspected. He told my mother that my grace and precision set me apart; my pointed toes and straight knees made me elegant amongst the other seven-year-olds. Still, this wasn't enough to become a Cabrielle.

There were prescribed tricks that had to be mastered before being promoted to the team. I still needed to learn the more difficult skills—a front handspring on the vault, a back walkover on the high beam—to be eligible. Leaning backward on the beam into the required walkover terrified me. The move was blind, and I didn't trust that my hands would indeed find the four-inch-wide wooden column, a harrowing four feet off the floor. My legs shook, my eyes welled, my heart pounded. What if my hands missed? I'd land on my head on the beam, then fall again to the floor. I refused to lean back without the feel of a spotter's hand at my back; just knowing it was there gave me the security I needed to lean backward into the unknown. By the time I flipped my body around—going from standing, to back bend, to handstand in the split position, to a stand again—the coach who had placed his hand at my back had stepped away and was standing clear across the room. When he refused to return to me, I'd hop down and practice on the low beam, positioned just inches above the floor. I'd make walkover after walkover on the practice beam and finish class without ever returning to the high beam. I couldn't bring myself to "go for it" despite the shaking knees and queasiness. With my fearful temperament, I'd never make it in gymnastics, Rich warned. I had to stop being such a chicken, he told my mother.

Quickly the praise of my first days in gymnastics class had turned to condemnation. When I was seven years old, gymnastics was already about what I *hadn't* learned yet, what I couldn't do, what wasn't mine. Just like my parents, so quickly dissatisfied with their first house in Cherry Hill, desperately wanting the bigger home in a more affluent neighborhood, near the well-to-do second graders I went to school with, I only wanted what was just beyond my grasp. Gymnastics was never about celebrating what I'd accomplished, what new tricks I'd mastered. There was no time for pride when there was so much to learn. I gently settled into the mode of striving, always striving, for what I didn't have.

# Chapter 3

AND THEN IT HAPPENED: I WAS IN-
vited to join the Cabrielles. Just before I turned eight, I'd
overcome my fear enough to learn the required skills and my
position was elevated from mere class-attending mortal to
competitive squad member. I'd get the blue warm-up suit
with the yellow block letters arced across the back, spelling
CABRIELLES. I'd wear a perfectly matched ribbon in my hair
every day, crowning my imperfect lumpy ponytail. I'd enter
competitions for a chance to win medals and ribbons. I was
proud that my hard work had paid off.

We practiced four days a week, sometimes five, for three
hours a day. I no longer attended the amateurish-sounding
"gymnastics class"; rather, I had "workout." With no article
preceding the noun, it made the whole affair seem really professional to me. Before, as a class girl, when I couldn't play after school, I told my friends "I have a gymnastics class today."
Now, as a Cabrielle, I mustered all the affected nonchalance I
could to simply tell my friends: "I have workout." I no longer

spent any afternoons at home watching *The Flintstones* and *Speed Racer* cartoons with my brother after school. Tuesdays and Thursdays had been free before I was a Cabrielle. Not anymore. Monday through Thursday, four o'clock to seven o'clock, I was in the gym.

Weigh-ins were required as a Cabrielle. Once a week I'd submit to the doctor's scale, positioned off in a dark corner by the bathroom. I'd try to sneak it in between turns on bars, pretending I didn't really care what the number was, that I was acceding to the process simply because I had to. Feigning nonchalance, I'd race through the procedure, tiptoeing on the scale's platform and scrawling my weekly number onto the chart that hung on the wall comparing our week over week heft. I'd speed through before a coach had the chance to look over my shoulder, notice that I sometimes subtracted a pound or two when I penciled my weight into the little box reserved for that particular week, just to ensure that Heather didn't beat with me with lower numbers. My mother didn't know we stepped on the scale once we became Cabrielles, and it didn't seem important for me to share that with her when I had more exciting updates about the new tricks I'd learned. But her own weight concerns—she often boasted of the cottage cheese and bologna diet that accomplished a mere ten-pound weight gain during her pregnancy with me—supported my developing theory that putting on pounds was to be avoided.

Some of the older girls, the Class Ones, were already developing curves. While my classmates in school anxiously awaited the day when they would get their first training bras, I knew this was something to ward off. Coaches whispered about not being able to "do it with the extra weight." I had enough trouble mastering the advanced skills; I didn't need fat thighs to provide another obstacle. Cindy Chiolo, one of the Class Ones who was already in high school, had hips and boobs that seemed to complicate things. She was always adjusting her bra beneath her leotard, fidgeting. The bounce of her chest appeared to slow her down. In between routines, she sauntered around the gym, talked of boyfriends and movie dates. I imagined that she was "easy" like Annette from *Saturday Night Fever*, whose well-developed body got her into trouble in the backseat of a car. After seeing this R-rated movie with my parents, I linked a developing body to danger and unwanted male attention. Cindy seemed to court these things. Her body seemed sloppy and uncontained, and so did her life.

I knew that wasn't for me. She wasn't serious like Linda. Skinny and athletic, Linda was the best girl in the gym. She made state championships. She could do a "full" on the floor exercise (a back flip with a full twist), the first in our gym. In 1977, that was something. Olga Korbut had won the Olympics just five years earlier with only a layout on floor and a back flip on balance beam. Linda could do all of Olga's tricks and more. She seemed impossibly mature, dedicated, and accomplished for only thirteen years old. I just wanted to be half as good. Heather was the one to beat because she competed in my age bracket, but Linda was the one I aspired to be. Just a few short months on the team and I brushed aside my satisfaction with the accomplishment to make way for a new goal. I would be as good as Linda.

When I joined the team, I was taught the Class Three compulsory routines, the first step toward competition status. I practiced them obsessively, at the gym, in my backyard, on the tennis court waiting for my mom to finish her weekend match. I couldn't wait to enter my first meet. If mastering these routines was the prerequisite, I would do it in record time. Competitiveness bubbled over in me. Wanting to compete—and win—was my greatest distinction.

There were no optional routines at this level, only

compulsories. These required routines were crafted by the United States Gymnastics Federation to demonstrate a girl's basic skills, those mandatory to be a competitive gymnast—technique, grace, and flexibility. They were the equivalent of figure eights in ice-skating. Optionals were routines designed by a girl's personal coach, devised to showcase her personal strengths—athleticism, poise, personality. They were dangerous, marketable routines that flaunted the sport's daring and the athlete's moxie. Today, these commercial sets are the only ones required of a gymnast; compulsories were dropped by the International Gymnastics Federation in 1996, dismissed as uninteresting to audiences and TV sponsors.

While we learned our compulsories, we were also preparing the more difficult tricks necessary for the Class Two level, when both compulsories and optionals would be required. Twelve to fifteen hours a week was deemed the appropriate schedule to master both the compulsory routines and more ambitious optional skills. It was also the amount of time required to instill a sense of discipline while blocking our view from activities competing for our attention. How could rapidly developing preteen girls be distracted by socializing, going to the mall, and hanging out with boys, if they never had the chance to see or experience them?

After school, I went right to the gym. We'd start with some stretching on our own while the ordinary class kids finished up their playtime. Heather and I would giggle and chat about our school day while we splayed our legs into splits and twisted our backs, cracking them for maximum looseness. She was now my friend, and we bonded while laughing at some of the class kids, the uncoordinated ones, flopping around on the floor trying to learn simple skills like cartwheels and forward rolls. These things came so easily for us, it seemed these girls just weren't trying. We'd talk about how much homework we had to do that night when we got done with practice, and sometimes Rich would interrupt us while we stretched.

"This isn't playtime," he barked. "You're on the team now." We had an obligation, as the representatives of this gymnastics club, to take our practices seriously.

"How many bridges did you do?" He pointed at me.

"Two or three," I mumbled. The remorse prickled, bringing heat to my face. I was not embarrassed at being caught. I was shamed. I felt untrustworthy. Contemptible. Lazy.

"Which is it, two or three?"

"Two," I admitted.

His eyes narrowed in condemnation. "And you?" He pointed to Heather but softened his tone. She was his favorite.

"Five." She lied with indifference. This separated us. Earnest in my desire to stand out, I'd go to any lengths to reap honest praise. Heather enjoyed a compliment even if she hadn't earned it. If she had to try beyond what was comfortable or easy, she'd lie to get away unscathed.

Pleased with Heather's response, Rich pointed at me again. "Stop talking so damn much. Make it five more. Like Heather. Before you start workout." He turned to the group. "All of you!" But he'd pointed at me.

Then, once the classes were dismissed, we'd gather our things—our gym bags filled with handgrips and beam shoes, our Thermoses filled with astronaut Tang—and begin our workouts. We'd rotate from one event to the next, an hour on each. Debbie, Rich's wife, was stationed at the balance beam. Rich was on tumbling. Marty, the assistant coach, always stayed positioned between vault and bars, shuttling back and forth.

We toiled to perfect the rudiments of the sport on each apparatus. Sometimes we'd get to mix in a little trampoline if we were learning a new tumbling skill for the floor exercise. We'd practice it on the "tramp," harnessed into a spotting belt, Marty standing on the floor pulling us up and down with a pulley, stringing us up like marionettes. We'd get our bearings this way, before having to embark on a skill solo. Good days were the days we got to do trampoline. For a young gymnast, it was recess.

The rest of practice was strenuous and consequential, from the very beginning. There were tears almost every day, either from physical pain or simple frustration. Or fear. Dread. Having to try the full twist for the first time without the belt or take the newly learned back handspring from the low beam resting on the floor to the *real* one four feet in the air. These were burdensome tasks. By junior high school, many of the girls I'd trained with were burned out. The daily fear of injury was an exhausting strain, and for many, it was just too much to take.

I embraced the anxiety-inducing training schedule. And it wasn't long after I joined Cabrielles that I went to my first Class Three meet. The only thing I knew of gymnastics competitions was the Olympics that I'd seen on television. I envisioned stadiums, cheering crowds. Perfect 10s. Gold medals. Prize money.

My dad dropped me off in my gym's parking lot with some money and a wave. He didn't usually drive me to the gym, but it was a Sunday and he was off from work. I climbed into the white van with all the team girls. My parents didn't attend the meet. They weren't allowed to. The Tobins frowned on it, claiming it made us more nervous, impeded our performance. Perhaps our coaches were showing some foresight, protecting us from our staunchest supporters.

I was gussied up for the occasion. I wore a navy blue pom-pom atop my ponytail. My hair was shellacked, Aqua Net crisp, to ensure bumps would not leak through midway into the competition. I'd lose points for that, I was certain. I proudly wore my team warm-up suit and felt like a real professional.

We drove the hour and a half on the turnpike to northern New Jersey. We climbed out of the van and entered a gym that was very dark and musty; it was subterranean. There were no spotlights or announcers, no cheering crowds. It was just like our gym, only gloomier. This was the first indication that I wasn't quite at the championship competition level that I'd daydreamed about on the car ride there.

We were permitted an hour or so to warm up. We stretched, then did a round of routines on each of the four apparatus. And then it was time to begin. I was nervous. My voice was choked down in my throat, as if smothered by a stone. My legs shook on the beam as parents sat in folding chairs near the baked goods, cramming fifty-cent Rice Krispies Treats down their gullets.

I went through all four events and fell on three of them. I fell three times on the balance beam alone. On vault, I took a tumble on the first attempt, hands and face smashed into the mat after my layout squat. On the second go (two turns on vault is customary), my vault was nearly flawless. Just one step at the end of a soaring, graceful coup would result in a nearly perfect score, I assumed. And then a 5.1 was flashed. My breath caught. That was lower than expected. Very low compared with Nadia. Tears of disappointment rolled down my cheeks. Then I reconsidered and pulled myself together. It was not such a bad score compared with the 3.1 I got on bars and the 3. something on beam. And it was on par with the score I raked in on my best event, floor exercise, the only event on which I remained upright the entire time, playing to the judges as I'd seen Nadia do on television. I even waved to the other girls' parents on the sidelines upon completion of my routine, as if an adoring crowd was giving me a standing ovation.

My total all-around score was in the neighborhood of a 15. About 50 percent more than the highest possible score for a single event. But my total had two digits. Many of the girls didn't even get to 10. They were sobbing in their mothers' arms, inconsolable. While my performance lacked the elegance of those I'd watched on television, and my scores lacked the dazzle of the 9s and 10s I'd hoped for, I now had a tangible goal. I aimed to get to a 20 in the all-around by the end of the season.

We drove home in the white van, cradling our winners' tokens, counting them over and over. Despite my imperfection, I won a few ribbons. They handed out the flimsy satiny kind that came in blue for first, red for second, and white for third. There were three more colors all the way down to sixth, a regal purple. My best place was third, on bars, for my 3.1. The stinky dank gym, the low scores, the absence of my parents in my shining moment, were eclipsed by the thrill of stepping onto the winner's podium—a makeshift step with three levels (places fourth through sixth stood on the floor, at the winners' feet)—and accepting my prize. That ribbon, which probably cost less than twenty-five cents at a local trophy-supply store, was pure gold in my hands. I stroked the satiny cloth, pride beneath my fingers. I'd brought home more ribbons than any other girl on my team. I was determined to win even more next time, to elevate my placements. Still, I was a bit confused; unclear on the distinction between professional and amateur athletics, I thought I was supposed to get paid for my ranking performance. Where was the winner's purse to go along with these ribbons? Too embarrassed to ask any of the older girls— perhaps I'd gotten it wrong—I contented myself with admiring my ribbons for the rest of the ride home.

When we got to the parking lot at our own gym, my dad was waiting to pick me up. It was late, but I was excited. I leapt from the van to show my dad the shiny, slippery evidence of the day's triumphs. He hugged me, proud, happy that I was happy. In the car, I offered up my change, a Rice Krispies Treat and a soda shy of the ten dollars he had given me before the meet. "Keep it," he said. "It's yours." I believed I'd won my professional payment after all. Tired and content, my pockets were teeming with money and the day's prizes. And for a fleeting moment, I was satisfied.

# Chapter 4

I LOVED PERFORMING. AND ONE OF the perks of being on the team was that we got to perform in exhibitions. Positioned to our parents as a way of breaking us in for competition, getting us used to tumbling for an audience and learning to manage our nerves, Rich would parade us around from shopping mall to amusement park to suburban swimming club, where we would spin and twirl for a handful of moms and kids. Before we went on, my legs turned to jelly and my breathing became shallow. Though I was racked with anxiety, once I was out there, I couldn't get enough of people oohing and aahing and clapping because of me. It was fantastic. The moms would see us looking cute as we smiled and tumbled, and they'd want to sign up their kids for classes, which was the real purpose of these traveling sideshows.

Upon arrival at the site, the coaches would lay down royal-blue folding panel mats in a long row. A crowd would begin to gather, interested in the unusual setup. A mini-trampoline and a big softer mat were set off to the side, prompting whispers among the collecting crowd: "I wonder what those are for." "What are they gonna do there?" Then the music was turned on, flooding the swim club or mall with a disco beat.

First we'd run out to the center of the mat—the tallest girls in the middle, the littlest ones on the ends—and take our bows, like peewee circus performers. After getting all jazzed up on the applause, we'd position ourselves in two long side-by-side lines. Now the little pixies, of which I was one, were in front. Glorious. I was front and center, where all the attention was. We'd tumble in pairs, for the easy stuff. Then we'd mix it up as the difficulty escalated, two lines on either end of the long row of mats, tumbling daredevilishly toward one another, crossing in the middle.

I was always paired with Heather. As the two smallest, we were first in line. And of course, we got the loudest applause. "They're so tiny. And cute!" gasped the crowd of moms and kids as we spun ourselves dizzy, doing rows of cartwheels and back handsprings. We'd work our way up to the most difficult moves. Back tucks, layouts, sometimes full twists with a spotter.

We performed these tricks on mats placed atop the cement at the Cherry Hill Mall or the uneven hilly grass of the Marlton swim club. These surfaces were always too hard, too bumpy, or too slanted. It was the late 1970s, years before children were obsessively protected at every turn. Childproofing was not yet a multimillion-dollar industry; parents had never even heard of outlet protectors, finger-pinch guards, or toilet locks to prevent drowning. Our parents never complained about the circumstances—they were so proud watching their daughters star in these talent shows. And we were resilient. No one ever got hurt.

Usually, by the end of the show, we drew a pretty decent-sized crowd. As we started flipping higher into the air, little girls eyed us from across the mall and dragged their mothers over to see what was going on, begging to be signed up for classes.

Rich announced each of our names and ages and the skills we were performing on a microphone. I lived to hear my name booming from the speakers, floating across the swimming pool, echoing in the indoor shopping center. I felt so important and accomplished. Other seven- and eight-year-olds weren't being announced at the mall, unless they were lost and trying to find their parents. "This is Jennifer Sey, one of our youngest Cabrielles. She's doing a round-off back handspring back tuck!"

I'd land with a hop and wave to the crowd. They'd cheer. God, I loved it. *Loved* it. I listened closely to see who got more applause. Louder, longer. Was it me? Or Heather? I was convinced it was her, because she was cuter and blonder and better. But it was close. I certainly got the second most. And usually we went together, as the two smallest. I took comfort in knowing that they were really cheering for both of us.

For the finale, the coach would pull out the mini-tramp with the fluffy mat behind it so we could really throw ourselves around. We'd run, hurdle, land on the mini-tramp, and hurl ourselves into the air, performing untold numbers of flips and turns. I'd always try to perform multiple twists, really wanting to win over the audience, establishing my superiority. Inevitably, I'd fall. I'd lose my bearings, eject from the twist midair, and land on my back. "Oh!" or "Ow!" the audience would gasp. I'd stand and wave, convincing them I was okay, that even if I wasn't the best, I was the toughest.

After the show, we'd get to stay wherever we were and play. If it was a swim club, we'd go swimming; if it was the mall, we'd eat at the food court. If it was an amusement park, like Great Adventure, where we went every summer, we'd go on the rides. Most kids visited Great Adventure at least once during their summer vacations, but for us, because we were part of the day's entertainment, the entry fee was waived. Our allowance money could be wholly dedicated to cotton candy and carnival games.

Great Adventure was also special because Marty, our assistant coach, performed as a diver there. After we did our first exhibition of the day, we'd go watch him fly from the high dive, soaring in tandem with other aging acrobats. He saved us front-row seats for the show, so when the dolphins emerged, balancing balls and catching snacks midair, we were called from the audience to touch their slippery skin and feed them fish. It was always the best day of the summer by far.

If my family was on a weekend vacation at the Jersey shore, I made my mother bring me back for the Great Adventure show. She did so willingly. She felt special having a daughter who had so many obligations; there was pride in having a child who drew so much attention. And though there was a feigned exasperation when she explained to her friends, "(Sigh) I can't today. I have to drive Jen to Great Adventure," she didn't want to miss the biggest exhibition of the year any more than I did. With all the summer foot traffic, we always drew our largest and most enthusiastic crowd at the amusement park.

Even with all the gymnastics activity—practices, meets, and exhibitions—I remained dedicated to ballet. And at eight years old, amidst the flurry of gymnastics activities, I earned the lead in my first recital. All of the gymnastics events had prepared me for the performance. Nerves simply weren't an issue. I played the principal girl mouse, wearing a satin pink tutu with white polka dots, black sequined suspenders, and ears like Minnie. I loved this costume. It made me the star. I sparkled in the front, all the other kids seemingly drab and unimportant in their matching, unadorned, unsparkly corps de ballet uniforms.

The recital was held at the Haddon Fort Nightly, the general gathering place for town happenings in Haddonfield. A stately gray building with regal white columns in front, it was generally reserved for town hall meetings, craft shows, and local symphony concerts. The auditorium seemed enormous to me. My parents sat three rows from the front, gazing up at me, smiling encouragement. When I appeared center stage for the first time, I took my position: right leg front, left leg back, toe pointed under, left arm raised gracefully above my head. I waited for my partner—the little girl playing the boy mouse—to hit her mark, but I couldn't see her beside me. After hearing the music cue our pas de deux, I turned to find her. Too far downstage, she'd failed to hit her position. While standing there adamantly in my pose, I waved her over to the appropriate spot. When she didn't heed, I simply told her what to do. "Move over! You're in the wrong place!" She scooted over and we finished our duet.

I assumed no one could see me directing her. I believed there was an invisible curtain obscuring the audience's view of the behind-the-scenes shenanigans, while allowing perfect vantage of the choreographed performance. But it wouldn't have mattered if I knew they could see me. It was most critical that she do this thing right. And it was my responsibility to make sure she did. So I simply told her what to do, and then everything was fine.

Of course afterward everyone laughed about how bossy I was. Miss Claire and my parents thought it was hilarious that I was so dictatorial at such a young age. My father chided me with not-well-concealed pride.

"You always have to be right," he said with a slow shake of his head and a cryptic smile beneath his overgrown mustache. Hadn't he taught me that being right was the most important thing? When he raised his voice and hurled a menu at my mother in a Chinese restaurant, wasn't he justified because he was right? Right about some inconsequential detail, but right nonetheless. And at that same restaurant, when he made me eat an entire bowl of hot-and-sour soup, to prove that I'd been wrong in asking for such a spicy, adult dish, wasn't he just illustrating that he was right once again? My mouth aflame from the spicy red pepper, I cried, complaining of a sudden stomachache, insisting it had nothing to do with the soup (because that would have made me wrong in asking for it). If being right was tantamount to winning, as he'd taught me, I'd do anything to prove my virtuousness.

Backstage at the recital, I vigorously defended my actions during the performance. "She was in the wrong place!" I insisted. It never occurred to me that I might embarrass this other girl by bossing her around in front of an audience. It had been my chance to showcase my talents as the preeminent dancer in the class. If my partner was fumbling around downstage, shuffling her feet, spinning in circles, she would have detracted from my winning performance. I felt I was the obvious champion of this recital. Everything was a competition to me, and there was no Heather vying for the number-one spot in this arena. It was just me at the top of this class, and everything had to be perfect to showcase my superiority.

My parents smiled an "I know, dear" smile as they handed me a bouquet of yellow roses. They looked at each other, shaking then bowing their heads with "What are we in for?" resignation. They could see it already. A competitor's ire was emerging. When I knew what I wanted, I'd sacrifice anyone who got in my way.

Though I was fiercely independent, a growing anxiety manifested itself in behavior at home that was considered immature and inappropriate. I refused to sleep alone in my room.

I was terrified. I had nightmares of witches and death. Deep into sleep, green-faced, hook-nosed hags surrounded me, cackling. A curled finger beckoned. I'd awake panicked and sweaty. Other times I'd dream of guns wielded at 7-Eleven stores, botched robberies resulting in *death to an innocent bystander, a young girl.* This is how it would be reported on the local news. In my dreams, I saw myself lying in the aisle of the convenience store, surrounded by soda and chips, blood draining from my body onto the tile floor, my mother huddled over me, crying. I was still alive, but I couldn't speak to tell her so. And, in my dream, I'd come to a terrifying realization. That was what death was. Conscious but unmoving. Unable.

I was told my great-grandmother "died in her sleep." I interpreted this to mean that death in sleep just happened. Add to that the fear instilled by the standard before-bed prayer, "If I should die before I wake . . ." and I was certain dying in one's sleep was common. The news shows, rife with local murders and other assorted atrocities—fires, car crashes, razor-blade-infested Halloween candy—fed into my obsession with death. Subsequently, I hated to sleep by myself.

While I toiled at the gym with the dedication of a professional athlete and directed entire ballet recitals, I reverted to near infancy at bedtime. I slept curled up next to my mom, teetering on the edge of my parents' full-sized bed. I had to sleep on her side because my dad didn't tolerate such nonsense. Despite the fact that he touted the "family bed" in his pediatric practice, he felt it had gone too far in our house. He created a little girl's utopia just across the hall, complete with frilly pink-and-white sheets, so that he could sleep comfortably, stretch his limbs, be alone with my mom. My mother let me sneak in with her, I suspect, because she enjoyed my needing her, my being a child, even if only in sleep. I cuddled next to her, warm and protected, shielded from sleep-induced annihilation.

One night my dad decided that enough was enough. He insisted that I sleep in my own room. He roared, unleashing his frustration with the uncomfortable three-to-a-bed arrangement. Bawling in desperation, I positioned myself on the floor outside their bedroom, on the threshold of their locked door.

"I hate you!" I screamed as I pounded and clawed at the door.

"Do you think she really hates us?" my mom whispered from inside the room. Her voice cracked with tears.

"Go back to your room!" my dad boomed.

"I'm scared!" I pleaded, snot running across my lips, salty on my tongue.

"She's still a baby," my mom cried, her whisper elevated to a plaintive whine.

He didn't succumb to either of our pleas. He didn't want to know why I was so scared and anxious; he didn't want to talk about it while patting my hand and stroking my hair. He just wanted me to sleep in my room. Sometimes a parent needs things that can obscure a child's needs, and he needed sleep. He snapped a belt from inside, threatening. My father didn't believe in spankings and encouraged his patients to discipline their children in other, less violent ways. He counseled them that intimidation was not the way to teach a child. But he lost sight of that in his exhaustion and frustration. The unfamiliar threat of violence sent me fleeing into my room. I slammed the door for protection, cowering but desperate to get out and back to the safety of my mom's cozy side of the bed.

Once things quieted, I tiptoed back to their door. It was still persistently shut. Each breath I took was cautious. I touched the door gently, silently begging to be let inside.

"Go!" he shouted, snapping the belt. He'd been waiting for me. He knew I'd return. He knew I'd need to be pushed to do the right thing, the big-girl thing. To be brave and set aside my fears.

I scurried back to my room, gasping for breath between sobs. Sleeping alone was unthinkable. I had to come up with another solution, so I snuck into my brother's room, positioning myself on the floor next to his bed. Chris giggled, threw his stuffed animals at me. My father heard and snuck up on me, through the bathroom that connected Chris's room to my parents'. He snapped the belt and I fled for the last time. In my room, I cried myself to sleep, too spent to dream of ghouls and dying.

I woke in the morning, exhausted from all the sobbing. There was a note beside my bed, propped on the nightstand that I'd spray-painted pink with my dad just weeks before. On the gray cardboard that his dry-cleaned shirts came folded over, he'd scrawled a letter in his illegible doctor's handwriting. "I'm proud of you. I love you. Daddy."

It was all I needed.

My dad's affection and approval tamped my foreboding angst, allowing me to endure the nightmares and distress. We never talked about why I was so frightened. From then on, I simply set the fears and anxieties aside, squelching anything that got in the way of my dad's validation. After that night, I slept alone, braving the horrifying monsters, witches, and real-life villains lurking just around the corner of sleep.

# Chapter 5

I WAS MATURING AS A COMPETITOR. The developing ability to overcome my fears in the gym and suppress my nerves during competitions was hastening my ascendancy in the world of New Jersey gymnastics. After a year as a Class Three, I did an obligatory stint as a Class Two. I qualified for state championships, where I performed admirably, hovering somewhere around the middle of the pack of forty girls. In 1978, as a Class Two gymnast, states was the furthest you could go. Many girls languished at the Class Two level for years, never overcoming the stress of competing. These girls ultimately tired of the sport and gave it up for the high school cheerleading squad, a low-pressure way to show off while drawing the attention of boys. I was nine, having done my one-season quota at this middling tier, and it was time for me to be promoted.

Marty, the assistant coach, was my biggest supporter. Throughout my career I would never be favored by the head coach, always the assistant. The less important coach, the second-tier teacher, the one who inevitably did not own the gym, always took a shine to me. Perhaps he saw me as the one with the second-most talent, the one through which he had the best chance of proving himself worthy. He couldn't have the most obviously talented as his pet—the head coach had dibs on that girl.

Blond and lanky with a wild look in his eye, Marty seemed crazy, albeit in an entirely lovable way to a nine-year-old. Though he was well into his thirties, he still demonstrated the gymnastics skills he was asking us to perform. This was endearing. Rather than shouting at us for being "chicken," he proved that what he was asking for was possible, even for an old guy who'd never competed on the balance beam (men don't do beam). And usually, the demonstration of whatever skill he was trying to elicit from us made us laugh. It just looked funny when a man did it.

Marty was the only male coach I ever had who had actually been a gymnast. Most of the male coaches of the 1970s and 1980s came to gymnastics either as a business opportunity (gym teachers capitalizing on the Nadia craze) or through an unseemly interest in being around little girls in leotards (gym teachers not satisfied with the privacy of interaction with students afforded them in the public schools). Marty simply loved all things dangerous. The gymnastics frenzy of the time gave him the chance to supplement his living as a gym teacher doing something more exciting than refereeing a game of dodge ball while providing him the means to pursue his own thrill-seeking adventures. He rode a motorcycle helmetless, storming into the gym's parking lot each evening, kicking up a cloud of dust. He competed as a cliff diver in Acapulco, garnering a slot on what was still my favorite TV program, *Wide World of Sports.* I watched him soar down along the majestic steep rock face, come dangerously close to crashing into the red escarpment, then slide into the water. If it had been the 1990s, Marty would have been an "extreme athlete," bungee jumping off bridges or double flipping his Motocross bike, turning high above the dirt piles in an X Games arena. He was an adrenaline junky with little regard for his own safety or dignity. He'd embarrass himself if it gave him a thrill.

Sometimes Marty would dress up in a leotard, hair in pigtails and bows, hairy legs poking out, crotch obscenely obvious. He'd perform at gymnastics competitions on all of the women's apparatus. He'd dance in a girly, humorous way, flicking his wrists and waving to the crowd. He'd straddle the balance beam, legs akimbo, face twisted into an exaggerated pained expression. He'd take to the uneven bars, spinning uncontrollably, round and round, unable to stop himself. On the floor exercise, he'd jackknife out of his trick midair, land on his belly and bounce on the springy floor, facedown and spread-eagle. He'd stumble to an upright position and finish the routine with a flourish and the pasted-on smile of a nervous little girl. We all laughed—the girls, coaches, and judges. He provided a humorous respite from the strain of competition, a break from our own less-than-perfect performances and the tears that went along with them. It was a reminder that this was supposed to be fun. Even the parents relaxed, chuckling in the stands, forgetting about how disappointed they were for their children. Or in their children.

In 1979, when I qualified for my first state championships as a Class One, Marty was there with me. He had been training me for the entire year, dedicating most of his energy and encouragement to me. Heather didn't interest him. She was talented but lazy. At this point, my four-day-a-week training schedule ramped up to five, Saturdays added to prepare for big competitions. Practices were at least four hours a day now, from three o'clock to seven. I don't remember fourth grade, but I remember preparing for states. The gym was everything.

As a Class One, I had to perfect compulsories and optionals. It was critical that I learn the more difficult skills to incorporate into my routines if I wanted to be a real competitor. I needed to include full twists and double twists on floor, Tsukaharas on vault (a half turn onto the horse, landing on the hands, a back flip and a half to land on the feet), back flips and tumbling runs on balance beam.

Marty was the one who encouraged me, helping me to overcome what Rich considered to be a prohibitive amount of fear. Even as I mastered the required skills, Rich consistently complained of my apprehensiveness to my mother. He used this to dismiss me as unpromising, despite my steady performance in competitions. Learning new skills took too much coddling, cajoling, and spotting. Rich had little patience or hope for me; I was more effort than I was worth in his mind. Though my mom never showed disappointment in me when Rich came to her with his grievances, she never put him in his place either. She never spoke up and said, "She *should* be afraid. Look what you're asking her to do!" She listened to him, respecting his position and expertise as the head coach.

Only Marty was accommodating enough to teach me and explain the mechanics of a trick. I had to believe in the physics of a skill before trying it. Without the *feeling*—a clear understanding of the way the skill worked—I just wasn't sure what would happen. And I had little faith that it would go my way. Perhaps I'd just sink to the ground, no momentum to spin me, landing right on my head. Perhaps I'd crash back into the bar—my head, a heel, my ribs colliding with the wooden pole. But Marty coaxed me, with verbal encouragement and physical assistance. I trusted him, and I'd try whatever he was teaching me if he stood close by, prepared to catch me if something went wrong. Over and over we'd do it this way, then he'd back away a little at a time, until finally I was doing it—a back tuck on beam, a flip from low bar to high bar—by myself.

At the Class One state championships in Summit, New Jersey, I performed any number of skills that I had been terrified to learn. A back handspring and a back tuck on the beam, a double twist on the floor. And bars. Nearly everything I included in my bar routine at this meet had traumatized me to learn. The straddled flip from low bar to high, catching between my legs, brought more tears and more crash landings than any other skill I'd learned to date.

We'd started the process of learning this basic release move (any bar move that requires letting go and then catching the bar again after some sort of flip) with Marty placing one hand on my back, one on my stomach, and carrying me through the trick repeatedly. For weeks, we'd do it this way. Then, as my confidence built, his hands hovered near me, not quite touching, grabbing at me in midair. If I missed catching the high bar, sometimes Marty couldn't pluck me from the air as I plummeted to the ground. He'd throw his arm between the floor and my back, softening the landing as best he could. If I made ten in a row with his hands near but not touching, he'd back away midtrick, until I was doing it by myself. Once I'd accomplished that, I was unstoppable, no longer afraid (of that trick, anyway). If I missed one, crashing on my back on the floor, I wanted to catch ten to make up for it. Learning tricks on bars was the most anxiety-ridden process of any of the events for me. That event rattled me.

But I nailed my bar routine at states. My only fall was on the floor exercise, where I overturned my second double twist at the end of my routine, bouncing outside the white lines for a one-tenth deduction on top of the five tenths for the fall. But it didn't matter. Most of the girls in New Jersey weren't performing double twists at the end of their sets. They were lucky if they could pull one off at the beginning.

My coaches warned against looking at my scores during competitions lest it instigate insurmountable discouragement for the remainder of a day, turning a meet from bad to worse. That year leading up to states, I often cried when I saw my ratings. Or when I finished a routine in which I'd fallen or bobbled or bent a knee that shouldn't have been bent. I cried a lot that year. In addition to fearfulness, tears were my attenuating weakness. While acceptable for children, tears were intolerable for competitive athletes. If I was going to "make it," it would be in only a few years' time. By twelve, it would be clear. Was I going to be nationally competitive? Or was I going to be relegated to state competitions and partial college scholarships at Division III universities?

Competitiveness offset my teary disposition, driving better-than-expected improvement in a short period of time. At Class One states, I scored anywhere from 8.0s to 8.9s on all my routines. Less than two years after my first meet, where I logged a grand total of a 15 in the all-around, I posted 8s on every event. I stood out at the state meet. I became a seasoned competitor. I looked at the scores and they galvanized me, propelled me to even better routines on subsequent events. Local coaches and judges started to notice me, to consider me as a potential talent. I exceeded their expectations, but they had underestimated me. In one year I'd gone from Class Three and 3s all the way to a regional qualifier at the Class One level.

Regionals were held in Silver Spring, Maryland. It was the first competition where I encountered girls from beyond the New Jersey state line. In addition to my fellow New Jersey gymnasts, Delaware, Pennsylvania, Maryland, Virginia, and West Virginia sent their best from the qualifying state meets. There were girls trained by nationally recognized coaches.

Lisa McVay from MarVaTeens and Maisie Chillano from Berks. These girls were clearly, without question, going to be the U.S. National Team members of the future. They would take the place of Heidi Anderson and Gigi Ambandos, of Kathy Johnson and Cathy Rigby. MarVaTeens coach Gary Anderson had put many girls on the national team. I was dazzled.

Somehow, with Marty's encouragement, I blocked out the other girls. I focused on doing what I did best: performing. My enjoyment of performing grew exponentially each year. Dreading the potentially disappointing results in no way diminished the joyful anticipation of competition and the absolutely addictive thrill of playing to a crowd, no matter how small. One judge was enough to get my adrenaline going.

By the time I got to my final event on the second day of regionals (compulsories were performed on the first day, optionals on the second), I had a chance of making it to sectionals. This competition would pit all the girls in the entire eastern half of the United States against one another. To qualify, I had to place in the top half at regionals. All I had to do was make my vault. I was doing a tucked Tsukahara. I rarely practiced it without a spotter, too afraid to perform it on my own in workouts. Marty was always there to help, to soften the landing, to catch me if I missed a hand. The only time I ever did it on my own was in competition, when the adrenaline was pumping.

Tentative but feigning confidence, I addressed the head judge. Given the stature of this meet, there was a panel of four judges on each event. The head judge acted as umpire, resolving disputes and calming irate coaches disappointed by low marks they considered unjust. The final score for each routine was an average of the two middle scores, the high and low ratings thrown out. I raised my right hand and pasted a smile on my face, signaling to the judges that they should prepare to take their deductions. My parents sat in the bleachers of the high school auditorium, with my aunt Jill and my brother Chris. It was all up to me. I shifted my weight nervously at the end of the runway. And then, my vision narrowed as I prepared to run toward the springboard, to sprint full speed down the vault runway, a skimpy rubber mat that lined the basketball floor. I focused on the horse and the board. Everything stopped. I had tunnel vision. Silence. I was in a vacuum. My focus honed to the point where I saw nothing but that horse and myself landing on the mat on the other side of it, fully upright.

And I did. I landed on my feet. Straight and proud. So lightly I almost didn't feel the impact. No steps. Perfect. I was walking on air.

With a pat on the back and a whisper of encouragement from Marty, I flew to the end of the runway to perform the same vault again, a requirement, the score, in this competition, an average of the two attempts. I wasn't out of the woods yet. I had to make the second one for a high-enough average to qualify. But now I was confident. I pictured myself "sticking it," landing without a step. It went beyond picturing it. I felt it. I actually felt myself landing on the blue mat on the other side of the horse. Landing, addressing the judge, making it to sectionals. Now it would be easy. I launched myself toward the springboard. I was light, buoyant. Practically weightless. I bounced like a beach ball, no impact, just fluttery bounce, floating down the runway. My feet were dragging behind me as my heart pulled me forward. I flew. I couldn't feel my feet on the ground. Pure adrenaline made me light, impossibly fluid. Like the air. I could barely feel my body, and yet I had perfect control. I did it. Just a slight step this time. But nearly flawless.

Marty swept me up in his arms, swung me around. I felt

like Nadia when Bela Karolyi lifted her in the air after her 10 performance on bars at the Olympics. Marty had always known I could do it. Despite my tears and tentativeness, he saw my determination. He knew I wasn't particularly strong or fast. I was a bit soft and lethargic for an elite-level gymnast. But I was tenacious. If I fell, I kept going. I tried again. If I couldn't do it one way, I tried another. I came first to practice, left last. And I didn't complain. I may have cried, but I never complained. Heather may have had more talent, but she simply didn't care as much I did. And now, I was the first and only girl from Cabrielles to qualify for sectionals.

Things were getting serious. Family time and recreational activities were no longer part of my life. I pleaded with my parents not to take me away from my practices, even for short family vacations, and they accepted the curtailment of these endeavors. Up until the point that I became a Class One, we'd spent extended summer vacations at the Jersey shore. I played stickball on the beach with my brother and dad and went to Million Dollar Pier for Skee-Ball, saltwater taffy, and the Guinness Book of World Records Museum. We'd gone to Mexico for Christmas the previous year, visiting Mexico City for museum culture and Puerto Vallarta for fun on the beach. We drove to a South Carolina golf and tennis resort on Kiawah Island for spring break one year, my brother and I crammed into the backseat of our midsized sedan for fourteen hours, my aunt Jill between us to prevent bickering.

Once I entered the world of competition beyond the state line, family vacations ended. And so did any memorable time spent with my brother. He was around but simply not a major player in my world. He came to all my meets, dragged by our parents, until he was old enough to insist on staying home alone. He'd taken up gymnastics at a young age, forced to fill the time when my mother took up desk duty at The Gymnastics Academy, checking class girls in during my workouts. He showed an aptitude, was more naturally daring and athletic than I was. But less serious.

I rarely attended his meets, my Saturday practices more pressing. The first and one of few that I went to was a chaotic three-ring circus. Little boys flung themselves from the high bar, spinning out of control through the air, landing on their heads, popping up without a scratch. One boy fell so many times off the pommel horse—the most difficult men's event—that he just gave up, walked away without finishing the routine. Acknowledging defeat, he sauntered over to his coach, who high-fived him anyway. Another boy ran down the runway approaching the springboard that would hurl him over the vaulting horse. When another boy crossed his path, the vaulter simply stopped, letting the interloper pass, and then continued his run.

Notably, there were no tears at this competition. The coaches didn't scream. The parents laughed and enjoyed their children. It was a very different picture from our meets. Or Little League baseball games, where parents and coaches seethed with rage at each misstep, every unfairness. In baseball—a little boy's sport—the dream of the major leagues was palpable. Olympic gold in gymnastics for boys just wasn't worth getting worked up about. Kurt Thomas, 1976 Olympic Team member, couldn't hold a candle to Reggie Jackson. The parents of boys in gymnastics had already made their position clear by choosing gymnastics. They weren't expecting much, they were just in this for a little character building.

And so for boys, the overall experience in gymnastics was less businesslike at a young age. Not only was the sport less vaunted for males, but the preparation required if a boy was serious (which presumably only happened if he was not very good at baseball) was quite different from that for girls. Because boys didn't turn into serious competitive gymnasts until they physically developed into men, their training ramped up more slowly. Their window of opportunity was wider, which allowed for less aggression and psychosis on the parts of coaches and parents.

Even though we both did gymnastics, I viewed my brother as a frivolous, undedicated boy, a careless dabbler. He did gymnastics, but he also dove and swam on the team at Erlton Swim Club, the local summer hangout. He had friends outside the gym and flirted with girls and took guitar lessons. He could only stumble through two songs—"Song of the Volga Boatmen" and "Yesterday"—but he pursued a variety of interests. He hadn't settled into a chosen path. He was a child, and we no longer had childishness in common. The more I got involved in the gym, the less like other kids I felt. I avoided the social situations in which my brother shined. His confidence and charisma seemed to grow exponentially while I became a better gymnast. We no longer spent time together because I was always at the gym. The fact that my brother continued to have fun both in gymnastics and outside of it, while I retreated into a very serious world devoid of play, created a divide. We just didn't share a life stage—childhood—any more. My focus became so narrow at such a young age that I don't remember much of anything but the gym.

# Chapter 6

MY SUCCESS AT 1979 CLASS ONE regionals couldn't be solely attributed to the Cabrielles' training regimen. As my intensity amplified, so did my mother's commitment to enabling my success. Her willingness to completely dedicate her time to securing the very best coaching and incremental instruction—chauffeuring me to and from ballet class, to choreographer, to Cabrielles workout—created the circumstances that allowed me to flourish. The additional outside coaching that augmented my workout schedule at The Gymnastics Academy was instrumental in my recent small but significant triumph.

The summer prior, I attended camp at the Parkettes club in Allentown, Pennsylvania. A national training center, Parkettes boasted many elite-level girls and former Olympians. For a week, I bunked with other hopeful gymnasts who wanted to be trained by the best. Bill and Donna Strauss, the owners of Parkettes, were ranked among the country's legendary gymnastics coaches. They developed Gigi Ambandos, Heidi Anderson, and Gina Stallone, National and World Championship Team members. They also coached young girls, up-and-coming stars, who were my age. Ten-year-olds Cindy Rosenberry and Nicole Kushner were already training for the elite level. The Strausses didn't compete these promising athletes at the lowest ranks. The Class One and Two circuits were considered remedial and beneath these future champions. Bill and Donna coached them until they were perfect, then unveiled them to the world in elite qualifying meets. Much like the Russians, they launched them at only the highest levels. Parkettes learned to be competitors not by competing, rather by training so hard they knew nothing but how to succeed.

After camp practice one day, the team girls performed. They flaunted their skills, flying across the mat the way we did in exhibitions back at home. But they soared through double back somersaults—two rotations in the air without touching the ground. Then each of them performed individual routines: triple twists on floor, multiple back handsprings and flips in a row on the balance beam, double back flyaway dismounts off of bars—they'd actually swing around the bar, let go when their backs were parallel to the floor, and hurl themselves through two somersaults before landing on the ground. On their feet.

Patrick, a scrawny, wild-haired assistant coach, taught the youngest girls, including Cindy and Nicole. These two were opposites—one blond, the other dark. One with perfect pin-curled pigtails like Cindy Brady, the other with a glamorous long straight ponytail and olive skin like a pint-sized Cher. Patrick admired them with an obsessive bent, drove them with an unyielding ardor. He shrieked obscenities when they failed to perform, slapping their bare legs if they paused before attacking a skill. He also hugged them with a lingering, unabashed indulgence.

Patrick taught my group during camp. I wanted to impress him, but I feared his disposition. Unlike Marty, he didn't accept cowardice or a tentative nature. Though I was generally afraid when taking on new tricks at Cabrielles, here I was without trepidation. My fear of Patrick translated into fearlessness when it came to attempting difficult new skills. With tremendous apprehension, none of it visible, I threw myself into dangerous new moves on vault, bars, and beam. My concerns about physical danger were completely eclipsed by my dread of experiencing Patrick's disappointment, something I never had to worry about with Marty. And while Rich often expressed frustration with me, he did it without Patrick's pronounced vehemence. Patrick's intimidating nature mitigated my cowardice. I was certain that, if I followed his instructions, he would lead me to perfection.

In addition to Parkettes camp, my mother employed a dance coach to hone my balance beam and floor exercise routines. Janet Cantwell was a former elite, a national team member in the late 1960s and early 1970s. She was one of several Cantwell sisters to compete at the national level. She now coached the University of Pennsylvania gymnastics team, an inauspicious assignment for someone who'd achieved such prominence. The Penn Quakers may have been scholarly Ivy Leaguers, but they weren't very good gymnasts. At age ten, I was better than all of them.

The university gym was old and run-down, not a gym where champions trained. It was airless and musty and ill equipped, stocked with shiny, slippery wooden beams, not the padded, slip-free variety that we had at The Gymnastics Academy. The bars were also wooden, nothing like the modern fiberglass kind that flexed, designed to give under weight, providing extra bounce and lightness. And the floor exercise mat did not have springs in it like the kind that we trained on, newly installed by Rich Tobin himself, to encourage more difficult skills—double backs and double twists. This equipment was hard and merciless, unbending and unhelpful.

In the late 1970s, gymnastics equipment had advanced to meet the needs of our advancing skills, to prompt us to greater heights and danger. The apparatus aided us, throwing us higher and higher in the air, egging us on, urging us to perform more and more impossible tasks. But this gym had given up on harder tricks. The equipment, held over from the earlier part of the decade, seemed hopeless and sullen, patient with those who'd lost their competitive edge.

Despite the woebegone setup at Penn, I went there twice a week for special instruction in dance for gymnastics. There was no hiding behind glossy equipment as Janet schooled me in the basics. She taught me how to stay on the beam, to bend my knees in order to bring my center of gravity back on top of the rafter rather than bending at the waist and grabbing at the beam to stay afloat (an ineffective and costly technique). She taught me how to finish moves with elite perfection, with grace and poise, flexibility, "amplitude," and extension. She prodded me to overextend my legs so there was no question whether they'd bent, thus causing a critical one-tenth deduction. She focused on the details that set regular girls apart from true competitors, from champions. Over and over, I'd practice the same dance moves—leaps, tour jetés, double turns, splits that went beyond 180 degrees.

She whispered to my mother after my practice that I was coming along nicely. She told her about another gym, close by, in Mount Laurel, New Jersey. The coach was Lois Musgrave, who was known for being kind but tough. Lois trained two elites already, the famous New Jersey elites, Suzie and Donna. She suggested Lois might be the coach for me.

Though Janet wasn't as obviously mean as Patrick, I was

also afraid of her. Somehow her stern glare, her silence, her obvious disappointment in my mistakes, inspired fear in me. I was terrified of letting her down, of not being able to do what she asked of me. She was an expert, a seasoned competitor. I believed if I heeded her direction and minded each detailed suggestion, I would improve. If I persevered, performing as many repetitions as she required, I would become a good gymnast, possibly a great one. If I handed myself over to her, I would achieve beyond my hopes and beyond my parents' expectations, which I sensed to be significant and growing at this point, given the financial investment and all the driving back and forth. In the days before "soccer moms" bought minivans, my mom was spearheading a movement of mothers dedicated to their children's extreme success. Not everyday, garden-variety accomplishment, but life-changing wins and breakthrough fame.

I believed if I gave in to Janet's instruction with complete abandon, adhered to her coaching with disregard for my own physical fear and emotional apprehension, I would not disappoint her or my mom. When she told me to practice a tumbling series on the hard slippery wooden beam that terrified me, I complied. When I missed a foot and slid down the side, scraping and bruising my leg, I jumped up and tried again. When a "raspberry" formed that burned and ached, I kept going. I would not find out what happened if she got angry. I would not find out what would happen if I disappointed my mom, who drove me to and from New Jersey to Philadelphia and back again. The pain wasn't nearly as bad as what the shame of their disappointment would feel like.

And not just *their* disappointment. My own. I would never be devastated by my own failure if I just did whatever Janet told me to do. I kept quiet and toughened my exterior, stopped crying so much. I seethed with a competitive spirit. At ten years old, my ambition bubbled beneath the surface, like vengeance.

After my session at Penn, before my practice back in Cherry Hill, my mom and Janet colluded about my next steps—what I needed to master before sectionals, who might be a better coach to take me to the elite level. They conspired about transitioning to Lois after this next milestone. It would be an easy move. I'd just pick up my things, put the year of Class One competition behind me, and move on to training for the elite level.

While they talked, I gathered my things from the locker room. Grown women—overweight, flabby, horrifying women—paraded around naked after their swim workouts and steams. Their veined thighs drew my horrified gaze. Their jiggly legs, drawn with varicose veins like rivers across their mottled skin, were terrifying to me. They weighed themselves, then plodded off to their lockers, slowly pulling on their tight clothes. Why do they weigh themselves? I wondered. They're fat. Knowing the number will not make that any more or less true.

I pulled my things together as quickly as possible, wanting to escape the haunted house of fat women. I fled to my mother, relieved to be among clothed thin people, even those with unarticulated but frighteningly high hopes pinned to me. My mom and Janet lingered, chatting about my progress and untapped potential. Then I was taxied to my next practice back in New Jersey.

Amidst all this training and special instruction, when I was getting quite serious about gymnastics, there was a book that consumed my attention. *The Best Little Girl in the World* was a novel about young Kessa, a ballerina with a dangerous obsession to be thin. She purged, starved, and implemented all sorts of tactics to maintain a perfectly skeletal physique in the quest for a never-ending childhood. These behaviors enthralled me.

I hid the book in my underwear drawer, enticed by its sugges-
tions, aware that I needed to keep it a secret from my mother
lest she start asking questions about my state of mind. "You
don't think you're fat, do you?" "You don't feel bad about yourself, do you?"

She might ask these questions if she discovered the under-
lined passages and folded page corners. The highlighted para-
graphs of self-loathing that Kessa battled when she felt she
didn't measure up to the other girls in her ballet class might
alarm my mother. She might pull back on all the extra instruction. She might realize that, though she didn't pressure me, her
support could be interpreted by a child as pressure. She might
want me to try life as a normal kid for a while. And though
my anxiety mounted as my training intensified, I wanted to
keep going to see what was possible. I wanted to see how far I
could get in the sport, and I certainly didn't need my mother
interfering.

But mostly I didn't want to worry her. I feared she would
discover the asterisks in the margins next to Kessa's tips on
starving and purging—eating one pea at a time during dinner, using a toothbrush to tickle the back of the throat. Then
my mom might concern herself with my emotional and physical health, torture herself with doubt and indecisiveness. *Should
I intervene? She's doing so well, that must mean she likes it. Dieting is normal, right?* I wanted to protect her from that kind of
distress. She seemed anxious enough driving me to and from
practice all the time. She didn't need to torment herself with
my secrets.

I felt about this book the way I would later feel about Judy
Blume's *Forever*. Like most junior high school girls, I memorized all the steamiest passages in this book, a tale of a teenager's
first love and subsequent loss of virginity. They delighted me
with titillating accounts of a first sexual experience. I tucked the

arousing stories somewhere private in my brain, knowing I wanted to try this stuff—not now, but definitely someday.

Weight loss and starvation would surely be required to build upon my successes, I surmised. Regionals was one thing—there were accomplished girls in that meet who didn't have lean, perfect bodies. Not so on television. All the elite-level girls were carved to perfection. If I chose to continue beyond sectionals, getting to the nationally competitive level would require me to go to lengths I hadn't even imagined yet. I knew Kessa's anorexia wasn't for me. Not now. But someday.

# Chapter 7   Qualifying for sectionals was a

turning point. I alternately daydreamed of bombing, missing every event in humiliating fashion, and winning the whole thing outright. The conflict between these two potential outcomes (not to mention all the other possibilities in between) created acute distress.

In the spring of 1979 I had a month until the meet. I'd had a full day of practice, first a session with Janet after school and then on to Cabrielles for a four-hour workout. I was readying myself for the biggest competition of my life. The meet drew the best Class One girls in the eastern half of the United States. I'd never trained so rigorously. I didn't want to embarrass myself in front of recognized coaches and future national team members.

After a tough workout, I sat in the kitchen of our new Haddonfield home. My father had managed an upgrade to our living situation, his new practice now thriving. We lived in the WASPy haven that my parents had aspired to as a "better place to raise children." Despite my elevated residential circumstances and the honor of participating in the upcoming, very selective competition, I was crying. Debbie had given me a hard time at practice about the new floor routine that Janet had choreographed. She chastised me, demanding that I return to her original choreography. Debbie and Janet had competed against each other as teenagers. Janet was the better gymnast, and it was likely that Debbie was now jealous that the nemesis of her youth was stealing her star pupil and throwing her choreography into the trash. So she took it out on me.

"Who do you think you are? You can't change what I did! Put it back!" She sounded childishly petulant. Her face was red, her bloated pregnant body imposing. I didn't think I had any choice but to obey this authority figure. But I knew Janet's routine was better, more intricate, closer to par with the national-level routines I would encounter at sectionals. I came home and cried to my mother. She flew into a rage, calling Debbie at home.

"You listen to me, Mrs. Debbie Tobin! She's my daughter, and I decide what's best for her! I decide!" My mother shrieked into the phone with animal pride and ferocity. She jabbed her finger into the air as if she were poking Debbie's chest, pushing her into a corner with a bullying thrust. Her jaw clenched, her eyes narrowed. She felt within her rights to ensure my success in the best way she knew how. If Debbie's choreography was uninventive, lacking elegance and style, my mom was justified in finding someone who could do a better job. She couldn't have me disappointed at sectionals, under-scored for performing an unsophisticated floor routine. Now she felt attacked for doing what she thought best for her child. And she wouldn't stand for me being punished in such a cowardly fashion. She felt Debbie should have come to her, rather than shaming me. My mother's ire was invoked in a way I'd never witnessed.

While she screamed into the phone, I sat with my head on the glass-topped kitchen table stifling sobs. At the time, I wasn't sure what she was so upset about. I wanted her to comfort me when I told her what had happened that evening during practice, not fly into a rage, calling my coach at home. Her outburst would surely prompt action. This exchange would require that I move on from Cabrielles. I would inevitably need to find another gym, leave my friends behind. How could I go back into the gym the next day? Debbie would scream at me during practice, hurling epithets and obsceni- ties while showering Heather with compliments, out of spite, despite the fact that Heather hadn't even qualified for sec- tionals. Rich would completely ignore me, sentencing me to hourlong conditioning sessions—pull-ups, leg lifts, laps around the floor mat—forbidden from practicing my rou- tines. Marty would back away, unwilling to get caught in the middle of the Tobins' marital collusion, a business decision to drive me and my disagreeable, demanding parents from the premises. This feud would be taken out on me in a humiliat- ing manner.

I'd never heard my mom scream like this. She rarely yelled at Chris and me. We were well behaved and generally went without major punishments. Arguments with my father were behind closed doors. He may have raised his voice with her, but she took it, saved her defense for later, when we were tucked into bed.

She wasn't one to assert herself. She was a stay-at-home, suburban mom, timid and small, barely one hundred pounds. Other moms we knew were choosing to go back to school, get their law degrees, become nurses, teachers, therapists, anything but *just* wives and mothers. These baby boomer women were empowered by the women's lib movement and the push for the Equal Rights Amendment; they sympathized with Meryl

Streep's character in *Kramer vs. Kramer*, when she left her young child and her husband to pursue a life of self-actualization—a previously unthinkable act. These other women gobbled up Betty Friedan's *The Feminine Mystique* and took to asking for divorces. Our friends' moms were dating, working, figuring out the intricacies of joint custody.

My mom chose us—me, my brother, my dad. And she wasn't in the habit of berating others to get what she wanted. Yet here she was, raging into the phone because she wanted something. *She* wanted something and she was going to get it. She stood in her well-appointed kitchen howling at my coach, in supposed defense of me. It was primal. Frightening. It was horrible.

I knew something was off. It seemed too important to her that I get the treatment she knew I deserved. This wasn't just about that day's practice, about Debbie getting mad at me about the floor routine. Because really, what did it matter if Debbie gave me a crappy floor routine to boring classical music? To *Cavalleria Rusticana*. (No one wanted to watch a pixie trot around to serious classical music. Little kids were supposed to have *cute* music, like a circus song or the theme from *E.T.*). So what if Heather got the cute routine, to *The Wizard of Oz*? And so what if they thought Heather was the better gymnast? Didn't this all start out as fun and recreation? Wasn't it still supposed to be?

But this wasn't just about the floor routine. This was about all the practices in which they'd shown Heather preferential treatment after all the extra effort my mother had put in. That investment, representative of her love for me, was being trampled, dismissed. Heather's mom didn't work nearly as hard for her daughter's success as my mom did. She went to the beauty parlor to have her hair dyed peroxide blond and the tanning salon to brown her leathery skin while Heather was at the gym. She didn't watch practice, work behind the desk. This was evidence that she did not love her daughter as much or, at the very least, did not have as much blind faith in her potential. In addition to defending my right for the best floor routine I was capable of delivering at sectionals, my mother was fighting for the title of best mom.

How could such fury be invoked if it wasn't *really* important, life-change-ingly important, future-hinging direly important? If my mom couldn't keep her head amidst all the craziness and competitions and ever-raising stakes, I'd better be good. I'd better be the best. She was going to make sure I had every opportunity to be, so that she could also prove her bestness. I promised myself not to let her down.

Things weren't the same after the argument. I begged my mom to apologize to Debbie, and relations were repaired sufficiently to get me through training for sectionals. The Tobins were civil to me in the gym, but it was a hostile civility, so I stuck by Marty as I prepared for the upcoming meet.

My family, coaches, and I flew to Atlanta, the host city, a few days before the competition. Debbie stayed home. Marty would coach me through the meet; Rich came along as the gym's owner and representative, with plans to strut around boasting and recruiting a bit while skillfully concealing his lack of authentic belief in me.

It was exciting. I'd been on a plane before—family vacations had taken me to Disney World in Florida, even Guadalupe and Mexico City. But I'd never traveled beyond a car ride across state lines for a meet. My family was hopping a plane and flying somewhere for me. Everyone—my mom and dad, my brother, and even my aunt Jill—was there. Some kids boarded planes and flew halfway around the country with their coaches; their parents were either trusting, busy with other family responsibilities, or unable to afford the plane fare.

But my immediate and extended family was deeply involved and supportive. This first meet established our family's routine. I would never travel anywhere alone. I would be girded with "Go, Jen!" cheers, hugs of support ("It's okay, Jen. You'll get 'em on the next one!"), and, of course, practical doctor's advice from my dad ("It's not broken; let's splint it until we get home!")

When we arrived in Atlanta, I had a day of practice at the auditorium before the competition. It was a gigantic arena, not a dark, musty hole of a gym reeking, of chalk dust and sweat. It wasn't a high school basketball court with makeshift bleachers. This was a real live competitive arena. A university stadium. To me, it might as well have been the Colosseum.

I was the only girl from my team at the meet. Heather had already proven herself distracted and undedicated, skipping practices and missing competitions in recent months. Her talent was no longer enough to keep her at the head of the class, and she hadn't even made it past states. And Linda suffered from Osgood-Schlatter disease, a painful knee condition afflicting girls undergoing growth spurts. She was out for the year. While I felt honored to be the sole representative from my gym, I wished I had a friend with me to experience the camaraderie of competing with a team, or at least a teammate.

By myself during the premeet practice day, I remember being awed by the other girls there. Some would go on to be national team members in the very near future. Lynne Lederer, scrappy and athletic, was from a prominent Chicago club, Mid-American Twisters. Rumor had it she could win the nationals and would definitely qualify for the elite level next year. Her coach, Bill Sands, also famously coached Amy Koopman, who was on track to make the Olympic Team in the upcoming year. No one doubted Lynne's ability to take this competition.

Another standout in the meet was from West Virginia. Mary Lou Retton was all power and dynamism; she could fly, jettisoning her stout, muscular body across the vaulting horse without the slightest effort. I was intimidated and terrified of being found out as not worthy of my spot in the competition.

Despite Lynne and Mary Lou's dominance, the most impressive girl there was Torrance York. Though these others were the best gymnasts, Torrance was the most famous. She had been featured in a book called *A Very Young Gymnast* by Jill Krementz. I had the whole series—*A Very Young Skater, A Very Young Dancer, A Very Young Rider*. But Torrance was my idol. And here she was. I was starstruck. She looked just like she did in the photos in the book. Lean, dark-haired, poised. I wanted to be her.

But it turned out she wasn't that good. I beat her and I was three years her junior. She fell to the very bottom of the eighty or so girls in the meet, while I lingered near the halfway mark. I managed to stay relatively calm throughout the competition despite the fact that I was overwhelmed and scared. I was one of the youngest girls there in the junior category (those under fifteen), and coaches noticed me. While I didn't qualify for nationals by making the top half, I performed with pride and self-assurance, missing it by only a few spots. I had only one fall—on bars, my perpetual nemesis. Strong vault and floor routines on optionals day brought me scores in the high 8s. Marty beamed. Rich hovered, arm around my shoulder, afraid I might wander off and find myself another club by the end of the competition.

Only recently, Rich wouldn't have cared if I left his gym. Now it became clear that I was the one with drive and quiet, gutsy ambition. I was the only girl at Cabrielles who was willing to sacrifice any semblance of a normal girl's existence to become a winning gymnast. I'd exhibited the qualities of a champion. I was willing to self-destruct to win. Other girls who cried as much as I did ended up quitting. I'd endure any amount of fear, come through it tearful and shaky, and keep going. Now that Rich had seen these qualities in me, he wouldn't watch me go without a fight. While he hadn't considered developing a club of national prominence when he started Cabrielles, he now saw possibility for his gym. And I was the one who presented that possibility of taking his little club from New Jersey obscurity to the national spotlight.

My parents began to wonder aloud where this could go. Just three and a half years earlier, I'd started gymnastics as a way to get some exercise. Though the sport had already eclipsed our family's recreational time—weekends were dedicated to practices and competitions—it had not yet fully taken over my life the way that it did for elite-level girls. I still went to ballet class with Miss Claire. I attended school full-time. I lived at home with my family. If I was sick with a cold, I stayed home from practice. I had advanced well beyond what was expected, but that just meant I had an aptitude, not a full-fledged talent. My skill was not yet deemed worthy of breaking up the family or risking health and happiness for. Up until this point, winning hadn't entered the family's consciousness. But suddenly, it was coming into focus. Seemingly mythical only a year before, it now seemed possible. A palpable and plausible consideration.

Only a handful of girls ever made it to the elite level. To me, that world was imbued with fame and specialness and a certain starry quality. I had heard girls talk about the elites. Janet told my mom and me about Will-Moor, located just a few more minutes down the highway from my current club, where two elite-level girls trained. Will-Moor's Suzie and Donna were famous heroines to young Jersey gymnasts. Once qualified for elite, girls vied for spots on the national squad, the World Championship Team, the Olympic Team. Girls at this level traveled the world, competing in China, Eastern Europe, South Africa. I imagined these remote locations to be earthy and unpolished but exciting. To my knowledge, only journalists embarked on such adventures. It was an enchanting prospect for a young suburbanite. Many girls trained as elites in obscurity, never breaking into the top twenty, top twelve (to make the primary national team), let alone the top six who generally competed in the major international competitions. But just down the road from us, Will-Moor had placed two girls in the upper ranks.

Suddenly, qualifying for the elite level seemed a feasible and worthy goal in itself. My parents figured I could skip gym class, lunch, and study hall at school to allow for a full day of training from two in the afternoon to seven o'clock at night. Five hours a day in the gym seemed like a good start to train for the elite qualifier, less than a year away. They proposed this to the Tobins, out of courtesy. They'd taken me this far, after all. The coaches balked. Though Rich had been initially seduced by the thought of taking his club into the limelight, he realized that he and his wife were most interested in running a recreational gym, profitable enough to support their growing family. They wanted a good team, but only insomuch as it attracted girls to their money-making class program. They would fight to keep me but only to a point. I was a marketing vehicle. They would not rework their schedule around me.

Rich and Debbie had brought me as far as they were capable. Even Marty, patient and supportive, couldn't usher me to the next plateau. My coaches didn't have the technical expertise to teach me the required skills. They had no system in place to allow for extra training hours, before and after a shortened school day. They had neither the discipline nor the desire to take me to the next level. The Tobins conceded: I was now too good, too ambitious, for them. It was time to move on.

# PART II

1987

I'm standing at the end of the balance beam. My right foot is pointed in front, rolling back and forth between the toe and the ball of my foot. My left leg supports me. I squeeze it straight, lock the knee to prevent it from shaking. If my leg shakes, I'll melt into the beam, never going for the dismount. I lock the leg to keep out the fear, the possibility of injury, the doubt.

I rock. Back and forth. Back and forth. Five times. Ten. I lose count. I start from one and give myself a fresh count of three. I get to three and I'm still standing there. I haven't hurdled toward the other end of the beam, thrown myself into the round-off, hurled myself into the air off of the beam, into my double back dismount. It's a new trick and I'm terrified. I'm waiting for a sign. The sign, the feeling that it is right within my body, a rootedness in the pit of my stomach that tells me I will land on my feet once I throw my body into this ridiculous maneuver. And the feeling doesn't come, so I keep rocking. I must wait for the feeling.

My coach is getting impatient. She wants me to finish up. I have two more events to practice after this. Mrs. Strauss screams, "C'mon, Sey! What are you waiting for! Jesus Christ!" She walks away, disgusted with my tentativeness. Some girls don't think, they just go. I've never been able to do this. I have to understand it first, then feel it, then believe I can do it. And then I can go. Otherwise I just rock, feeling off kilter and ill at ease. Wobbly.

I start my count over. I make a deal with myself. If I go on the count of three, I can have two tablespoons of Diet Cool Whip after my nonexistent dinner of iceberg lettuce with vinegar and diet soda. I entice myself with artificial, low-calorie sweets, sinful ten-calorie faux sugar my just reward for going when I'm scared. And then it clicks. On my second rock I know the third will be magic and I will feel squared and centered, confident. I will rock a third time and go.

I shift my weight to the back leg and then lean into the hurdle on my front right foot. I feel unshakable. I am locked into the beam, melded to it, heavy and sturdy as a car on asphalt. I belong on this balance beam. I cannot be tipped or rattled from this perch. I place my right hand down, shifting the weight seamlessly from my feet to my hands, turning my body upside down. The left hand hits and I keep moving. There is no stopping now and no reason to. I push off the beam from my handstand, snapping my legs down, feet landing on the end of the beam, the left just slightly behind the right to ensure they fit on the four inches. My chest snaps up, I jump, but not willfully. It all just happens now because I've committed to the trick. I am nimble, breakneck precision. I am in the air, hurled from the end of the beam, spinning in a ball. Two times around. A double back. A much-needed new dismount to increase my difficulty for the upcoming championships.

I see the floor when I am upside down, release my body from the tucked position, and land without a step, intrepid in the knowledge that I can do this trick. And I can have a bite of fake dessert after dinner.

"Again, Sey. Ten more without a step."

I exhale, then climb back up onto the beam.

Each time is a process of convincing myself I can do it. Each time, I must overcome the fear of terrible neck-landing injury. Each time is an entire workout in itself, ten seconds of overwhelming panic and gut-wrenching despair. And courage winning out in the end. I live this process each day, twenty, thirty, one hundred times.

The fear never abates. It is constant, relieved only in the instant I have landed on my feet. It surges again and again and again. Agitation and fright is my perpetual state of existence. But I ignore it as I climb back up onto the beam and begin rocking.

1980-1984

# Chapter 8

I was ten years old when I began to inflict pain on myself to relieve a constant and growing uneasiness. When I started to compete in earnest, I also started gnawing at the inside of my mouth. I'd begin the whole process by running my tongue over a patch of wet skin just inside my lip. If I did it consistently enough, for long enough, the patch would turn red and sore. Now the nibbling could begin. I'd peel away layers of skin with my teeth. Once a blister formed, the chomping could begin. I'd chew my cheek until huge pus-filled blisters formed. My lip would then swell with greenish yellow bulbous cankers. On the eve of one state competition, I chewed so hard and so long that my bottom lip swelled to twice its size. Protruding, thrust outward, I couldn't explain it to my parents or my coaches. What happened? they asked. You must have a cold. I shrugged as I tried to fold it inside my mouth. It was too big. I couldn't hide it.

Once fully formed, round and glorious, I'd run my tongue over it. Again and again, for days at a time. The sore became hot and smooth. Constant irritation made it bigger, angrier, more swollen. The tongue was only a vague irritation. If I really wanted to feel it, I'd dig my teeth into it. Right into the center, as hard as I could. The pain would shoot through my lip, down to my chest. I'd hold it there as long as I could. It helped me to forget about the meet. While I was waiting to go, and my heart was racing, and my nerves were getting the better of me, I'd simply bite down as hard as I could. Piercing the hot sore until it bled or until tears welled in my eyes. Until my heart stopped pounding.

I also began to pull at the skin around my fingernails, the cuticles. I'd tear at the skin, hard from the drying chalk. My skin was so dry I could pull big chunks without peeling the skin beyond the piece I was after. It didn't peel, it came off in hunks, leaving holes. Or I'd peel newer, fresher skin down to the first knuckle, leaving my fingertips to glow red from blood and irritation. While I waited my turn at the chalk dish, dizzy with fear about a new trick I was trying to learn, I'd tear and tear. It never healed. I'd dig into one finger until there was nothing left to pull. No more hard, dry skin. Just soft bloody tender second skin. And then I'd move on to the next finger. By the time I got to the last one, days later, the first was healed enough to start again. And the chalk ensured that the skin dried hard and crusty, not soft and unpullable. Perfect. Distracting but not disabling.

This habit was easy enough to hide from my mom. If I kept my hands in my lap, tucked between my legs while we drove to practice, while we watched television at night, my mom would never discover my jagged, raw fingertips. She wouldn't have to ask my dad to intervene in matters linked to my physical and mental health. She could continue to focus on how to help me achieve my ever-elevating goals in gymnastics without facing my escalating disquiet.

Intensifying anxiety was outpacing my ambition, and I worked hard to keep this fact hidden from my parents. If they discovered it, I believed that they would curtail my training, intervening in my single-minded devotion, my dream of becoming an elite gymnast.

In the spring of 1980, a few weeks after sectionals, my parents and I made the decision to move on to the next phase of my gymnastics career. When my mom told the Tobins that we were leaving, they struck back with vindictiveness. They said we were starry-eyed. That, while my performance in the last year was surprising and seemingly promising, they knew that I was merely an industrious child with a competitive spirit. We were pushing too hard. We would end up disappointed.

But my parents were committed to the notion that I was a girl with unlimited potential. This was undoubtedly influenced by the fact that they knew I was bright. I excelled in school, mostly because I was so obedient I never failed to do exactly what the teacher asked. And while intelligence does not usually prompt athletic excellence, obedience comes in handy.

I was barely eleven years old, and I was recommending myself for a promotion. Lois Musgrave's gym, Will-Moor Gymnastics in Mount Laurel, New Jersey, was the obvious choice. It was just a few towns over, between Willingboro and Moorestown, and just a short half hour drive from our house. And Janet's endorsement made the decision easy. I was grateful not to have to relinquish my family life. Many girls and their families would make the decision to move clear across the country—to California or Oregon—to pursue their gymnastics careers. We simply had to drive up I-95 to Mount Laurel.

My first day at Will-Moor, my mother parked in the lot and

we walked in together, holding hands. I was nervous. I didn't know the girls or the coaches. I was accustomed to being one of the top girls in my gym. I was afraid I'd be one of the worst gymnasts in this new club. Even if I didn't embarrass myself with an inferior skill set, I was afraid of how strenuous and serious the training would be. I wondered if I could handle the rigor.

My mother had called Lois (soon to be known by me and my family as Lolo) ahead of time to tell her that I wanted to join her team. Lois had seen me at states that year, though she didn't compete her qualified girl due to unexpected injury. She was hoping we'd call, she'd told my mother on the phone. Without hesitation, she invited us to visit without any pressure to join. She wanted parents and girls to feel at home, like the club was a good fit for their family. Just come and check it out, she'd urged.

I was greeted with open arms and enthusiasm. Lois waved me in with a hug and said, "Let's get started!" I hadn't expected to work out that very day. I thought she'd quiz me on my readiness to train seriously so that she could make a decision about whether to take me on. I didn't realize at the time that Lois accepted all girls. You didn't need to "qualify" for her gym. She viewed Will-Moor as a safe haven for little girls who loved the sport of gymnastics. She believed the sport was simply a launching pad, best used to transform young girls into confident adults. And sometimes these same young girls could become great competitors along the way.

I loved Lolo from the first. She was warm and grandmotherly, almost fifty when I met her. She had three children of her own, all grown and involved in the gym in some capacity. But she had hundreds of kids in the gym who she loved like her own. She wore her hair in a sassy Mia Farrow pixie cut. She was short, barely five feet tall, and muscular. Physically strong, she was like no other grandma I knew. Despite her age and diminutive stature, Lolo still did a lot of spotting. She guided the little ones through new skills, gently steering them, protecting them, as they got their bearings. Her enthusiastic, always optimistic approach to coaching set her apart in the world of nationally competitive gymnastics. She clapped her hands, fingers stretched like a child. Her eyes glowed, actually twinkled with pride, when a girl learned something new. She jumped up and down when any girl was excited about her performance. Whether the routine was perfect or just improved, whether the girl was one of Lolo's or not. And she always had a hug. She hugged girls she was just meeting, she hugged girls who learned new tricks and those who struggled to master them, those who won competitions and those who placed last. She hugged parents. She hugged the siblings of her girls ("my girls" as she called us). She hugged us all.

The Tobins hadn't been particularly unkind. They were aloof, cool, rarely mean. They just didn't care that much about any of us. They wanted competent girls who competed at the state level so that they could use their Cabrielle team as a marketing vehicle to grow the class roster.

The other coaches that I'd come into contact with were neither as distant as the Tobins nor as enthusiastic and loving as Lolo. Those most decorated—the ones who led nationally prominent teams and coached Olympians—were notoriously aggressive and mean. The founder of a nationally prominent West Coast club was rumored to hit his girls. Girls talked of how he slapped his gymnasts' thighs when they didn't stick their beam routines during practice. It was an urban legend of sorts, but one that aspiring gymnasts held to be true. Every other girl knew someone who knew someone who'd trained there, experiencing the abuse firsthand. Bill Sands of the Mid-American Twisters exploded during competitions, unleashing his frustration when he felt his investment had been squandered due to a careless fall on the beam or a stumble on the floor. Tears invoked further rage, taunting him with weakness. It was whispered that the Strausses—founders of the Allentown Parkettes—withheld food from their gymnasts; many girls boarded at this nationally competitive club, unprotected by parental proximity. They were punished for weight gain—as were their adoptive hosts—with emotional abuse and name-calling. These notorious coaches had no patience for mistakes or tearfulness or an extra half pound. They wanted to win and nothing else mattered. They took on the demeanor of those Eastern European coaches who trained the world's best. They aspired to Bela Karolyi's greatness, confident that if they mimicked his approach, they'd produce girls as perfect as Nadia. And even though Béla appeared joyful on television, swinging Nadia around in celebration of victory, he was known to be despotic on the training floor.

Lolo was unique in that she had one of the best clubs on the East Coast, yet she retained the warm and nurturing demeanor of an elementary school teacher. Despite coaching girls to the highest level in U.S. gymnastics, Lolo remained loving and kind, vigilant about her influence in young lives.

At Will-Moor, I began training for the elite zone meet immediately. The qualifying competition—"zones," as we called it—would take place in less than a year. I didn't have a lot of time to learn the new compulsory routines and craft new optional sets that included all the required difficulty, but Lolo believed I could do it. For the first time, I had a coach who really thought I could become a great gymnast.

As a gymnast, I was similar to Lolo's star pupil, Suzie Van Slyke, who was already competing at the elite level. Ranked twentieth in the United States, she was tall and graceful, known for long-limbed litheness and ballerina poise. I watched her leap and dance across the balance beam in utter amazement. She was the gymnast I could aspire to be. I possessed some of those same qualities—grace and poise—in miniature, little-girl form.

Then there was Michelle Krupa. Suzie's opposite, she was gruff and trashy. With bleached blond hair, roots always showing, Michelle was muscular and crude. Lacking technique, she made up for it with scrappiness. She was Sylvester Stallone in *Rocky*. Michelle did gymnastics by sheer force of will. She was also preparing for the zone meet, her first elite qualifier.

Donna Mosely, Lolo's other elite star, had already ceded from the gym by the time I arrived. She competed one year at the elite level and then gave it all up for a normal high school existence. For Donna, the promise of Olympic gold was not nearly as enticing as the junior prom. She wasn't ranked high enough to make the 1980 Olympics that year. She'd have to continue training for another four years for a shot at the Games. So she gave up, the lengthy training too demanding to endure. But she didn't leave without inspiring a legacy. Angie Denkins was Donna's neophyte disciple. Donna and Angie were both black, unusual in gymnastics, where the top girls were always white and perky in bouncy pigtails.

Angie was destined to become my best friend, my fiercest competitor, my alter ego. She was my age but my absolute opposite. She was compact, all muscle. Not sinewy lean muscle but bulky weight-lifter muscle. Her thighs bulged, her calves popped, her biceps were like Popeye's. Her muscles sent her flying, speeding, soaring. She had never competed before at any level. She was being "saved" by Lolo, to be unveiled to the world at the zone meet the following spring. Lolo and the other coaches at Will-Moor clasped their hands in witchlike delight when predicting the awed faces of the judges seeing Angie for the first time. They would be wowed.

Angie was all power. She ran faster than me (than everyone), was stronger than me, was fearless. She could already perform double backs on the floor (two somersaults in the air), giant swings on the bars, handspring fronts on the vault. These were skills performed by Olympians. And Angie.

Although Lolo loved me from the start, appreciated my talents as unique and special and promising, Angie would always be more talented, more gifted. But she would also prove lazier, less driven, less able to handle pain, injury, any kind of setback at all. My "second-best" status in my early training had given me emotional strength. When no one was looking, I toiled. I improved. I didn't let not being in the spotlight, not drawing all the attention, stop me. I kept working—on my own, with help from assistant coaches. (I was destined to draw the attention of the assistant, Wes, at Will-Moor as well.) My second-bestness drove me forward, always giving me something to strive for. And I wasn't striving to reach the level of that "best girl." I was striving to beat her. To knock her down, kick her ass, take her trophy. And I would do it stealthily. I was the tortoise. I was never the hare.

My mom became integrally involved in Will-Moor as soon as I started. With every step I took toward the national spotlight, with every bit of increasing intensity, my mother followed in lockstep. While she wasn't active in the PTA at school, she was central to the informal collection of moms who aided in the day-to-day functioning of Will-Moor. They fund-raised, they worked the front desk, they handled minor first-aid crises during practices. My mother became a permanent fixture behind the front desk, checking girls in for classes. Her friends were the other moms of the girls who spent long hours in the gym.

She hung out with them in the waiting area, gossiping about who hadn't paid their bills that month.

It started casually enough, just helping out when they needed someone. But it quickly became an almost full-time job. It allowed her to be close to her children. At this point my brother's continuing interest in gymnastics had led him to Will-Moor as well. He began training on the boys' team when I joined. Though Chris had been happy at The Gymnastics Academy, if I went to Will-Moor, he had no choice but to go there, too. Our practices overlapped, mine extending on either side over his. It placed our family—me, my mom, Chris—at the gym for the better part of nonschool hours. From about three o'clock in the afternoon to eight in the evening, we were there.

The gym was our family's center of existence. Either Chris and I were there training, with mom working the desk, or we were driving to meets on the weekend, or pitching in to raise money for the gym's booster club, which helped to pay competition and travel expenses for girls who could not afford them. For my mom and me, everything started and ended at the gym. Chris participated in this dizzying schedule of events but without the same obsessive tendencies. He had no choice but to take part, really. If I was at the gym, he was at the gym. So he made the best of it, making friends and training with a lighthearted, enterprising attitude. What choice did he have? Who would've driven him to soccer practice or Little League with my mom squared away behind the desk, busy greeting class kids and directing them to the locker room?

My dad was on the periphery of the whole affair, as he was hard at work to pay for all of it. His Philadelphia pediatric practice was thriving. He kept it open six days a week, with 7:00 A.M. office hours as well as evening appointments for single working moms who couldn't bring their sick children to see him during the workday. He saw patients, managed the staff, paid the bills, ran the payroll. He was an attentive doctor and an industrious small-businessman. Nonetheless, he stayed involved in my gymnastics, attending all the meets, asking about the exhaustive details of my practices at dinner each evening. We always gathered together for family dinner no matter how late we all got home. But through it all, he maintained a life outside of the whole gymnastics whirlwind; he gardened in the backyard, went fishing on the weekends, read countless books while hidden away in his study. He maintained an inner life, apart from the family and the travails of competitive gymnastics and Will-Moor. His private thoughts, his free time, his personal priorities, were his and his alone.

But the gym took over my mom's life as it took over mine. It was her work, her friends, her family. It was her happiness. She wasn't there to merely facilitate or observe as some moms were. She didn't drop us off, then drive off to sell real estate or attend a class. She didn't start her own business or go back to school for a graduate degree. She made the gym her entire life, and she did it all willingly, enthusiastically, in fact. It gave her a sense of purpose that she'd never known. And while her sense of purpose was balanced with my own, it was also proportional to the overbearing emotional strain that I felt, manifesting itself physically with perpetually bloody fingers and fat lips.

## Chapter 9

THERE WAS AN OLYMPIC BUZZ IN the air. The U.S. hockey team had recently triumphed over the Russians in the 1980 Winter Games. They were celebrated as heroes, paradigms of scrappy determination. Guts won out over technique in the Lake Placid ice rink, proving that America was indeed better than Russia, on the ice and in the world at large. Angie and I were embarking on our first step toward Olympic possibility in training for the zone meet. Though 1980 wouldn't be our year—besides being too young to qualify, we were nowhere near good enough—1984 was a faroff, hazy opportunity. We loved the sport. Everything about it—learning new tricks, competing, the speculative promise of notoriety—was magical.

At my house, Angie and I watched the Olympic Trials—the competition that would decide the gymnastics team for the upcoming Summer Games, to be held in Moscow. We rooted for our favorite girls to make the squad. I cheered Tracee Talavera, the surprising young up-and-comer who wowed the audience with her outrageous beam routine. Angie loved Julianne McNamara, a whiz on the uneven bars; she spun like a whirling dervish, so fast she blurred.

Shortly after we celebrated the appointment of the U.S. Olympic Team, President Jimmy Carter declared a first-ever U.S. boycott of the Games in response to the Soviet invasion of Afghanistan in 1979. Carter had called upon the Soviets to desist from further aggressive action in Afghanistan. He required withdrawal by February 1980 and threatened that refusing to do so would result in endangering athlete and spectator participation in the upcoming Summer Olympics. When the ultimatum was ignored by the Soviets, Carter called upon the International Olympic Committee (IOC) to move the Games to another city, preferably Athens. The IOC rejected the request, and the U.S. Olympic Committee voted to boycott the Games. Carter went so far as to pledge to revoke the passports of athletes who planned to attend the Games without a team, backing his boycott with the force of law. The United States' political statement engendered the support of sixty-four other nations, which also boycotted the Games. The Moscow Olympics were attended by only eighty countries, the lowest number in decades. The USSR won eighty gold medals, almost two hundred medals in total. It was deemed the most lopsided Olympics in history.

Many athletes were devastated. They had trained their entire lives to compete in the 1980 Games and now, due to political forces they thought to be outside the realm of sport, their lifelong aspiration was thwarted. Three American gymnastics team members—Tracee Talavera, Julianne McNamara, and Kathy Johnson (twenty years old at the time of the boycott, ancient for a female gymnast)—would persevere four more long years, to compete in the 1984 Games in Los Angeles, the consummate realization of a dream.

Angie and I were traumatized. Somehow our future spot on the team seemed at risk, the sport tainted by the ugliness of the outside world. But we continued training. Our big meet was only nine months away. And now the elite ranks were bound to be packed in 1981, not thinned by the attrition that an Olympics usually incites. The girls who had made the team, and even those who just came close, would not drop out. They would press onward for another shot at gold, silver, or bronze.

The 1980 Olympics also marked the last time the existing compulsories, in effect since 1977, would be performed. Postsummer kicked off a new set of routines that would need to be mastered by those embarking on their elite career and those continuing beyond the disappointment of the boycott. There was a clinic in California led by one of the choreographers of the floor routine and a handful of prominent national judges. As an elite hopeful, I was shipped off to San Francisco to learn the sets. I went with Jan, an assistant coach at Will-Moor. Gym-teacher stout with long hair and lots of split ends, Jan was stoner-mellow, very seventies in her look and her outlook.

I was sent to California because I was considered the mature, smart one. Never the most talented, always the most intellectually able. Lolo assumed that I was the best equipped not just to remember the routines but to bring them back and teach them to Michelle and Angie. Suzie would have been the obvious choice to go, but at sixteen, she found herself wanting to follow Donna's departure into the pursuit of typical teenage desires. She had grown four inches over the course of a few months and was struggling with the sport. A growth spurt always creates particular challenges for a female gymnast. A taller, postpubescent body can make it difficult to perform previously mastered skills. More weight, more length, and more curves create more resistance in the air, causing awareness to go topsy-turvy. The new body is lost in space. Some girls adjust and others give up. With her recent growth spurt, her burgeoning body, and her beautiful face, Suzie was drifting away from gymnastics and toward boys. She was a sophomore in high school with a stunning face and the legs of a starlet. The boys were surely lining up, and their appeal was greater than that of the competition floor.

I was in sixth grade with no interest in boys or any life outside of the gym. I couldn't understand how Suzie could want to stop now, when in my mind she was surely a contender for the 1984 Olympics. I thought she'd have plenty of time for boys and parties when she went to college. But she knew that she'd already achieved her full potential. She'd gone as far as she could go in the sport and was satisfied. I couldn't comprehend this attitude of resignation. She was as close to an Olympian as I'd ever known. I thought, When you're that close, why stop? What's four more years for a lifetime of acclaim? But Lolo had instructed Suzie to take a break and figure out what came next for her—gymnastics or the life of a typical high school student. Either was fine. Gymnastics was Lolo's tool, used to build confidence and strength of character. Her gravest failures occurred when a young girl's self-esteem faltered and she became lost in self-destructive behaviors. Missing out on first place, quitting the sport—these were just fine with Lolo.

With Suzie out of the gym, Lolo seized the opportunity to give me some exposure to the national gymnastics world. If I was going to be a part of the cutthroat national scene, the influential judges and coaches at this event would need to know my name. Gymnastics is not an objective sport. As in figure skating, scores are doled out by judges who always have a personal bias that colors their view of a performance. It's not like track and field—there's no finish line to cross first. The sport is filled with politics—who you know, who likes you. And if a gymnast is well regarded, she will always get the benefit of the doubt from the judges when they are debating whether to take that extra tenth. Did she bend her knees? No. She couldn't have. She's _____!

I was honored to be selected to attend the clinic. It was an illustrious assignment—bring back the elite compulsories, teach them to the other girls. The first day at the northern California gym, I huddled amidst the other gymnasts, packed onto the floor exercise mat watching the choreographer, Mary Wright, demonstrate the dance moves. Intimidated but determined to glean all that I could from these sessions, I pushed my way to the front, as close to Mary as possible.

Mary was the assistant coach at SCATS (Southern California Athletic Team), one of the best teams in the country. Led by Don Peters, the SCATS were the preeminent team during the early 1980s, before Bela Karolyi set up shop in Texas. (Bela was already famous for being Nadia's coach; he would go on to coach Mary Lou Retton to 1984 Olympic glory.) All the best girls ended up at SCATS—Olympic team members Tracee Talavera, Julianne McNamara, and Kathy Johnson—even if they didn't start there. At the time, Don and the SCATS coaches trained more national team members than any other U.S. club.

And in keeping with the tradition of top coaches, Mary instructed with a stern edge. Her chubby body was graceful, her Australian accent charming. But she was scary. On occasion she would shriek at Becky Rashoff, the gymnast assisting her, demonstrating the routines. I was surprisingly bold. Though I was one of the youngest, and definitely the least accomplished, I pushed to the center-front position, focused on learning the routines. And on occasion, I stood out. When Becky faltered and Mary squawked, I was asked to demonstrate a leap series. Mary asked my name and waved me toward her, pushing Becky aside. Wide-eyed, I pointed to myself. "Me?" She nodded. I threw myself into the split leap, thrusting my legs well past 180 degrees. "*That's* a split leap!" she jabbed at Becky. Proud, I did it again as everyone whispered, "Who's that?" Jan winked in encouragement from her folding chair on the sidelines.

In between learning the routines, Jan and I explored the tourist attractions of San Francisco. We had ice cream sundaes at Ghirardelli Square, clam chowder at Fisherman's Wharf, and I bought iron-on T-shirts for my family at Pier 39. I chose one for my brother that I knew he would like: a SAN FRANCISCO rainbow decal. It was more glamorous than those we had admired on the boardwalk in Atlantic City, just a year before when we still took family shore vacations in the summer. It was much better than the matching Bee Gees shirts we already owned. I bought him other trinkets as well—Ghirardelli chocolates, a cable-car replica—wanting them to make up for my special status, both in the family and outside of it. I had an unconfirmed but creeping sense that he might be developing resentment toward me. My offerings placated my own sense of guilt more than they appeased him. But he was only seven, and gifts can go a long way toward forgiveness at such a young age. I was exonerated.

And exhilarated. At age eleven, I was traveling to California with a chaperone, getting myself noticed by some of the best coaches in the country. I buzzed with confidence as I began to understand my strengths during that week in California. I was graceful and flexible. And I presented myself with a maturity beyond my years. At the clinic, other girls my age had been called out to demonstrate tricky maneuvers that required brazen intrepidness, but I was the only fledgling young gymnast distinguished by composure and dignity. Over the course of my gymnastics career, I would learn to play to these strengths, using them to elevate myself above the rising tide of acrobatic dominance. A sport once called artistic gymnastics was now simply gymnastics, the *art* piece less important than ever before. While I made the most of my talents, I would fight to overcome my weaknesses—modest athletic aptitude, average strength and quickness, and disabling fear.

My weaknesses were never more pronounced or called out to me more blatantly than when Gary Goodson came to our gym. Which he did, not long after my trip to California. Goodson was a traveling consultant, a self-proclaimed gymnastics guru, who came to Will-Moor two or three times a year for special training sessions. He was balding and angry, and being mean to young girls seemed to be his calling. We usually took off from school and practiced for an entire eight-hour day when he descended. In anticipation of his visits, I always chewed a nickel-sized hole into the side of my mouth; it inevitably grew to the size of a quarter by the time of his departure. He put the fear of God in me. With a nervous laugh, my mother called him Gary God-son, then sent me into his lair.

Goodson brought all the latest state-of-the-art techniques to us, straight from Russia and China. His notion of the sport was all power, athleticism, and acrobatic difficulty. The other nuances of gymnastics didn't matter to him. He wanted wind-up dolls that could spring their taut bodies into the air performing unprecedented flips and twists. This put me in a precarious position.

After my triumphant return from San Francisco he immediately foiled my encouraged demeanor. He called me Dough Girl, as I lacked the muscular physique of his favorite, Angie. He told Lois and my mother, while I stood right next to them, "If she's lucky, I can help her get a college scholarship." I had already set my sights on the national team.

I cried uncontrollably when I got home that night. My mother tried to console me. "What does he know," she said.

"She does have kind of a bigger butt," my dad said, confirming my dough-girl status. He leaned back in bed, burying his nose in a *New Republic* magazine. "She's never going to have that build like Angie." I eyed my butt in the full-length mirror in my parents' room. It was kind of spread out, not tight and high like Angie's horselike hindquarters. I hadn't noticed until my father corroborated Gary's assertion. The tears welled as I stole away to my room, where I clutched my Holly Hobbie dolls and cried myself to sleep.

But I didn't give up. I went back the next day, more determined than ever to learn his half-baked techniques that were intended to enhance my speed, give me quickness that would propel me to new heights and levels of difficulty. We spent hours learning to run. He claimed to have spent months with Olympic track coaches, learning the ways of speed. He also claimed to have spent weeks with "the Russians" mastering the rudiments of tumbling. We toiled for days with Gary, perfecting round-off back handsprings that would allow us to project ourselves into the cutting-edge tumbling moves—double layouts and full-in backouts—that he insisted were required. But only with the basics perfected would we be able to perform these tricks, he avowed.

He used his approach to try to break me. He was the self-appointed gatekeeper, allowing girls to move on only when their mastery of the basics met his standards. He rarely allowed me to advance beyond the building-block skills to the culminating moves. My lead-ins—the round-off and back handspring—weren't strong enough, he insisted. While he may have been concerned about my safety, I felt he hated me and wanted girls like me thrust from the sport. He had no time or interest in gymnasts who weren't the embodiment of machinelike Russian athletic superiority. Of course Angie was perfect, always permitted to move on to the "big tricks." There was a vindictiveness in the way he pointed out how far ahead of me Angie was. He seemed to enjoy rubbing it in when he'd stop my practice to point out just how talented Angie was. He'd glare at me with a "see that!" look. His menacing grin said "You'll never do that." And so the buoyancy I'd acquired on my trip west was squandered. I was easily convinced of the things he said because deep down, I believed these things about myself.

My entire childhood was plagued by thoughts of subparness. I never felt good enough. Just one notch shy of perfection, one slot shy of number one, and I withdrew into a state of self-hatred and shame. Ironically, growing competence usually amplified the self-criticism, my guard against complacency.

I attended an experimental private elementary school in Philadelphia. We learned in an open classroom, at our own pace. That meant I took to my books to teach myself algebra in the sixth grade. I struggled with the $x$s and $y$s in the puzzling quadratic equations. I had no sense that most kids wouldn't take this on until high school. I fixated on the fact that I couldn't do it now. And I hated myself for not being able to fly through the unassigned homework. I pulled my hair, yanked at my cuticles, and chewed at my mouth while I sharpened my pencils in a last-ditch effort. The failure swirled inside my head, bursting forth as tears of frustration.

After dinner and dishes—not completed until eight-thirty, due to practices that stretched later and later into the evenings—I would pull out my algebra book to begin wading through the self-assigned problem sets. My dad always sat patiently with me at the kitchen table, intent on remembering ninth-grade math and coaching me to find the answers on my own. He toiled with me until the eleven o'clock news beckoned him, content for three short hours to occupy a helpful place in my life, outside of my mother's purview. Over and over, we'd practice the math problems, his undivided attention lavished on me. I'd cry. He'd hug me, brush aside the eraser dust, and we would start from the beginning.

Fed up with the ravaging nighttime battles I was waging with my homework, my mom marched into school to talk to my teacher, John (because it was a liberal hippie school, we called our teachers by their first names). She wanted to know why I struggled so with math. Eyebrows raised with surprise, he told her that I excelled. Not just in math, but in all school subjects. He knew that I was hard on myself. He explained to my mom that he'd urged me to slow down, take it easy, but there was no stopping me. My mother learned that I put all this pressure on myself to master the algebraic equations. I waded through the math book at my own pace, pressuring myself to succeed, wailing in utter vexation when I hit a wall. No one had instructed me to go so far, to take on algebra. I was the one who had insisted on forging ahead. There were no external requirements, no adults egging me on. No one was disappointed in my performance.

It was me. I was my own tormenter.

# Chapter 10

IT WAS TIME. THE SUMMER OF 1981, and I was ready for my first elite zone meet. I had trained hard with Lolo for a full year in preparation. Since the beginning of sixth grade, I was excused early from school to train for five hours a day. My liberal-minded school encouraged self-actualization and free expression, so they willingly curtailed my academic schedule to support my quest of qualifying to be an elite gymnast. And in my mom's usual fashion, she did what was required. She chauffeured my brother and me to school from south Jersey to Philadelphia every morning. She returned to pick me up in the afternoon, carting me back to Jersey for practice. Then over the bridge again, back to school for my brother, who was released after a full day.

That year, I trained hard, but I had fun. Angie and I became friends. We weren't yet official competitors, as we hadn't attended a meet together, hadn't been pitted against each other, racing for the higher rank. Before the zone meet, we were allied in our crusade. But I was envious of her—of the ease with which she learned new tricks, the most difficult of skills. She flew through double backs on floor, release moves on bars, full-twist Tsukaharas and handspring fronts on vault. I struggled with each of these, mastering them eventually. But it always took me longer, and it never came without inordinate effort, tears, or injury. Nothing came easily. On a tired day, I couldn't perform any of the challenging skills, even if I'd nailed them the day before. I had to feel strong and "on" to complete the swing, to land on my feet after spinning through the air off the vaulting horse, one and a half flips around. If I was fatigued, I'd only manage one and a quarter flips, resulting in a "thud" as I landed flat on my back. Wind knocked out of me.

Angie just soared. Over the course of that year, she'd perform one or two vaults during each practice, landing so lightly she practically bounced. Then she'd sit around complaining of sore bunions, icing her feet. I'd toil, one vault after another. *Thud. Thud. Thud.* While she watched, rebraiding errant corn-rows while she rested on the sidelines.

In August, we trekked to some gym in northern New Jersey to contend for a spot at the upcoming junior nationals in New Mexico. The juniors were those girls under fifteen, not old enough to compete in the Olympics. Despite the significance of this competition, the host gym suggested little import. It was a dusty, hot warehouse. No bleachers, just folding chairs for the parents.

No matter. The inauspicious surroundings had no bearing on the zeal and sense of consequence I brought to bear. I harnessed the adrenaline buzz and performed the skills that usually gave me difficulty with ease. Some girls were thrown by adrenaline. The ultrasonic energy, the seemingly drug-induced speediness sent girls reeling, jostled them from the beam, caused them to overshoot their tumbling runs and land on their butts. They lost their footing with all the acceleration. I found it focused me and gave me just the right amount of energy to fly. At the meet, I stuck my front handspring front vault. I made about one out of five in practice. At the meet, not a step. I swung from the bars effortlessly. My giant swings were better than in any practice—arms straight, torso and legs outstretched, flinging in circles around the bar, the body like a spoke in a giant invisible wheel. Angie and I, in our lime-green leotards with white polka dots, were the surprises in the competition. Who were these two pixies? I sensed it whispered by the judges.

Midway through the meet I realized I belonged there. I knew I'd qualify. I went in thinking I'd be lucky to make it to nationals in Santa Fe. Obviously, Angie would go. I never had any doubt about that. But during the course of the meet, I came to know that I was a strong competitor and I deserved my berth among the elites. I qualified without a struggle. Michelle faltered, failing to make the cut that would send her to senior nationals. But I eased right through it, along with Angie. My parents couldn't believe it. They were steady in their commitment but unsteady in their belief. With all of their support, they were never sure if I'd come through when it mattered. They were truly surprised at the end of the event that I had mustered the wherewithal and weathered the nerves to qualify for the next level.

I wasn't surprised. And neither was Lolo. Together we were steadfast in our belief that I could do whatever I set my mind to.

In the fall of 1981, amidst the country's excitement over the confirmation of Sandra Day O'Connor as the first female U.S. Supreme Court justice, I was on my way to my first national competition. Women and girls were moving up in the world. Thanks to Title IX, passed almost ten years prior, young girls grew up knowing that they were guaranteed equal access to any and all educational programs at the high school and college level. The law required that males and females were afforded commensurate opportunities to participate in athletic programs and enjoyment of scholarships. While Angie and I didn't know about the law, we felt its influence; we never considered ourselves "less than." Never considered that we couldn't achieve whatever we wanted to——in athletics or beyond.

With this empowered sensibility, I traveled to Santa Fe for junior nationals, along with Angie, Lolo, and Wes. True to form, I'd drawn Wes's attention, as he was Lolo's best assistant coach. He preferred me to Angie because of my work ethic. Angie complained of aches and pains or simply refused to try another set on bars or beam. The one under her belt was always good enough to satisfy her. I persevered until I thought whatever I was practicing was perfect. I was tireless, no matter what the struggle, and Wes matched my commitment each day of practice.

Of course, my parents and my brother went to New Mexico, too. The whole gang hopped a plane in support of me. Over the course of the next seven years, I would never travel to a competition alone. Supporting me would become a family obsession.

The first day—compulsories—I performed respectably enough, floating somewhere in the middle of the pack, just above the median. On my second-to-last event on the second day, I was on beam, almost through with my routine. No falls. I'd had a few shaky wobbles but nothing too egregious. This event was often a girl's undoing. Even the best girls, when unnerved, could fall more than once off the beam, taking the mandatory half-point deduction, thereby plummeting irrevocably in the standings.

I set up for my final tumbling series. On the first back handspring, my middle finger landed on the beam bent under at the first knuckle. I stopped, not performing the second in the series, jarred by the discomfort. Despite the pain, I persevered, continuing with my routine. When I next saw my hand as I struck a pose, I noticed that my finger looked broken, bent oddly at the knuckle. Crooked and stuck. And it was bleeding, dripping down my hand. I panicked. I had to get off the beam. I buzzed through the rest of my set, dismounting in a haze. Upon landing (with a great big step backward), tears escaped, then escalated to sobs on the sidelines as I fell into Lolo's arms.

I held the arm of my mangled finger at the elbow, bloody digit on display. My dad came running down from the stands. He examined my hand and told me that my finger wasn't broken. He explained that when I'd bent it under on the back handspring, my nail popped out from the bed, pulled away from the skin and was now unattached and dangling. It would need to be pulled off if it didn't fall off naturally. Uncomfortable, but not dangerous, I found it to be an embarrassing first competition injury. I'd drawn attention to myself crying as I left the floor, and now the diagnosis lacked the dramatic import that my tears had suggested. Humbled and slightly ashamed, I recovered quickly. My dad popped the nail back under the cuticle and taped it up, sending me on to my last event. Once it was bandaged, I could barely feel it, and I performed my floor routine to a medley from *A Chorus Line* without flinching.

The top six girls on each event qualified for a third day of competition, the individual event finals. Top scorers were awarded the medals for each of the events. Despite my injury, I was close on floor with a seventh-place finish. My double back had been flawless, my dance moves more sophisticated and elegant than that of most of the twelve-year-olds in the meet. But one place beyond the cutoff relegated me to the stands, while Angie competed on vault. I was envious of her accomplishment, but I tried to shrug it off. I didn't want to humiliate myself further with a jealous tantrum. I pretended all was fine, making the most of the free day while Angie had to prepare for the evening's competition. I explored Santa Fe's bazaar, replete with Native American arts and crafts. I bought a pair of pink moccasins and a knickknack, a coyote howling at the moon. Then I enjoyed a root beer float with my dad at the diner on the town square.

That evening, I sat in the stands, a spectator, cheering for my teammate. I didn't sit with my family. I sat with the other girls who failed to qualify for event finals. They all wanted to see my purple fingernail and splinted malformed middle digit, which I held proudly in the air as explanation of my nonqualifying status. I made the most of my time expelled from the competition floor, enjoying nachos while politely clapping for our fellow adversaries. I may not have won any medals, but I made some friends and found a sense of camaraderie amongst the girls at the bottom of the pack. In the end, I would be the only one of my newfound allies who would continue to compete into the senior ranks throughout the 1980s. Tenacity was half the battle in gymnastics, attrition a resolute competitor's closest friend.

Though the finger thing seemed a trivial injury, and it was, I began to develop a reputation at that meet as a tough athlete. Amongst gymnasts, judges, and coaches, I was considered a girl who could deal with pain, a girl who finished no matter what. I placed thirteenth out of about forty girls. I was in the top half. Not bad for the assistant coach's pet with a mashed-up finger.

# Chapter 11

ON A GOOD DAY, WHEN INJURIES didn't rankle, being in the gym was like flying. I felt invincible, not held back by the typically assumed constraints of the body. The flying wasn't what most people would imagine. It was never the flipping-through-the-air part. It was the being on the ground but feeling weightless and suspended. I could tumble across the floor, land a bar dismount from heights of over ten feet, and never feel the floor beneath my feet. Never feel the impact. Gliding across the floor, landing from the height of a single-story rooftop, I would land as softly as if I'd just stepped from the curb. My bones and muscles were loose and wiggly, held together, barely, by my skin. My joints bent past what seemed possible. I slithered, floated. I never felt creaky. My body's center of gravity was so squarely anchored, falling was impossible. I was rooted to the equipment. It was part of me. Walking the beam was like walking on the ground, effortless and natural. Descending from great heights was like bouncing on my parents' bed, soft and cushiony upon landing. I could will my body to do anything on those days, though I could barely feel my own limbs. I floated through the air, across the balance beam, spun around the bars. I was otherworldly.

On a bad day in the gym, my body felt off from the start. I could predict these days from the moment I woke up. On these days, even my skin pained me. When the alarm sounded and I opened my eyes, the first thing I did was test my hands by closing them. Sore hands didn't bode well for that day's practice. Often my hands were sore or torn from too much friction on the bars the day before. If they hurt when I woke, I dreaded the day. I knew that simply touching the bars would be excruciating, swinging around and around would be nearly impossible. If I stepped out of bed and felt my ankles throb as my feet hit the floor, it was confirmed. My familiar daily workout would be something to get through, not delight in. It would be all I could manage not to hurt myself. Completing my routines without flagrant error or learning something new was out of the question. On days such as those, upon awakening, I felt palpable fear. A bad day at the gym for a gymnast was never like a bad day in the pool for a swimmer. My times wouldn't just be slower. I knew the danger was real. It was possible that I would land on my head, break my neck. I could, conceivably, die.

I could only hope that I wouldn't wake on the morning of a competition knowing it was a bad day. I would not be able to find my center of gravity. Hopes of a strong performance were out of the question. On bars, I merely prayed not to hurt myself, to fall gracefully, without advent. Making a routine without falls was unthinkable. Staying on the beam was precarious. Not at home on the four-inch-wide, four-foot-high plank of wood and padding, it was all I could hope for not to fall three times during a routine. My feet weren't firmly planted on these days. My body was lost in space. I didn't know myself.

But the good days were worth holding out for. They brought a feeling of looseness and freedom and euphoria, of being more than alive. On good days, I felt invincible.

I went to junior championships in October hoping for a good day at the competition. My family accompanied me to Reno, Nevada. Teammates from home gave me quarters to play the slots for them. It seemed perfectly sensible. I'd play their quarters in the slots, as if in the video arcade, and they'd get a piece of what it was like to qualify for the most prestigious junior gymnastics competition in the country.

Angie and I visited all the child-appropriate attractions in Reno. We saw a live lion caged at the MGM Grand, and we played Skee-Ball at Circus Circus. I did sneak onto the gambling floor to play some of those quarters and was promptly escorted off. The guards were used to us. Little girls had been scurrying about all week.

During one of the warm-up practices, a girl from a Nebraska team, Traci Hinkle, landed on her head in the throes of a tumbling run. She descended from great heights, unfurled her body from its tight, jackknifed position as she lost her bearings, and landed—*Crunch*—on her neck. The coach railed at her, before even checking to see if she would or could get up. "What are you doing! Get up!" he raged. She stood, shook it off, tried the move again, as prompted by her coach. We (Angie, Lolo, and I) were all thrown, speechless. Why wasn't he concerned? Why didn't any of the adults—coaches, judges, trainers—intervene? Lolo went to her, to make sure she was okay. Traci waved her away. There was fear in Traci's eyes. Fear of the coach pressed her onward. She continued practice and everyone assumed she was fine.

On the first day of competition, we ceremoniously marched out onto the royal-blue floor mat, competition-style (a bit like a Nazi goose step). We took our places, as instructed, in a line from tallest to smallest. Each girl placed her hand over her heart, puffed with nationalistic pride, as "The Star-Spangled Banner" blared. Midway through the anthem, the line of girls parted from the middle with gasps and "Ohs!" I moved back as the line peeled away and saw Traci on the floor in a puddle of her own vomit. She was rushed to a nearby hospital, treated for a severe concussion. We proceeded with the competition, skirting the slippery puke spot on the floor, never acknowledging its significance. It was a joke—"Don't slip on the vomit!" one teammate said to another as she marched out to perform her floor routine.

At this meet, I placed thirteenth again, solidifying my rank in the top twenty junior girls in the country while proving that consistency was indeed my greatest strength. Though my performance couldn't have qualified as a euphoric *good day*—I wobbled on beam, struggled on bars—it wasn't a bad one either. And, most consequentially, I felt like a part of something. I knew all the girls. Angie and I befriended the other stragglers, girls who were there alone without teammates. (There may have been two of us, but we were stragglers, not part of an intimidating crew brought by one of the top three clubs.) We snuck out for ice cream and watched the Russian trapeze artists at Circus Circus with the other lone gymnasts. I didn't have these kinds of friendships in school; leaving each day a few hours before classes ended singled me out as an oddball.

I also knew the judges. And they knew me. As I was warming up on bars, I missed a move and muttered to myself, "Fuck!" As I rechalked my hands, an influential judge, Audrey Schweyer, winked at me, laughing. "Don't say that during the meet, Jen," she joked, calling me by name. She caught me, but we were friends.

My parents had gotten to know the other parents as well. One dad who knew my father was a pediatrician asked, "Dr.

Sey, how can I keep Barrie from getting her period? She's growing so much faster than the other girls. It's going to hold her back." Always quick with the retort, my dad quipped, "Get her pregnant." Not the answer Mr. Muzbeck was looking for, though he chuckled anyway, perhaps alerted to the absurdity of his question.

We were in. The entire Sey family was a part of something that made us feel uncommonly accomplished, enjoined in our mission to enable my success. We were a team dedicated to a single player's performance, confident we would all be extolled and enjoy the spoils of that player's victory.

After the meet, we celebrated. All the competitors received tickets from the hotel to go see Bill Cosby perform. We all knew him from Saturday-morning cartoons as the voice of Fat Albert. I was familiar with some of his more mature material because my parents were avid comedy-album listeners. While they often spun records by Monty Python, George Carlin, and Richard Pryor, Bill Cosby was their favorite. Before placing one of his albums on the turntable, my dad always told a story about visiting my mom at Temple University when Bill Cosby was a student. He insisted that Mr. Cosby performed impromptu stand-up in the cafeteria in the days before he was famous. My dad said that he'd hop up on the lunchroom tables, practicing his jokes and stammering comedic style while the students watched, incredulous, over their grilled cheese sandwiches and tomato soup. In our house, Bill Cosby was legendary. It was an honor to be invited, the first inkling that being special held certain privileges. None of the girls in the meet would have missed this for anything. Even Traci Hinkle went, head bandage and all.

I sat in the audience with Angie and the other gymnasts and experienced heartfelt camaraderie as we laughed in unison in the dark. In my chicest outfit, a satiny, red, Asian-inspired jackety thing, I was on top of the world. Here in Reno, with a bevy of girls from all over the country, my friends. I felt so worldly. Then, as if it couldn't get any better, Bill called us all up onto the stage. "I understand the junior national gymnastics squad is here," he said in his best Fat Albert voice. He sounded just like him. He was him. We all looked at one another in amazement. "C'mon up here!" he crooned.

In a perfect line, we all descended upon the stage. I felt undeniably famous as I stood there, swanky and young in my Chinese jacket. And then he started asking us questions.

"What place were you?" he asked Traci, her bandage capturing his attention.

"I didn't finish."

"Huh. I shoulda guessed that." He moved on to the next girl, unceremoniously. "And you? What place were you?" he asked.

"Sixth," girl two replied proudly.

"Yeah. Now we're getting somewhere. Why aren't you wearin' your medal?"

"I left it in my room," she whispered, barely audible.

"What?" he pounced.

She shuffled her feet, too embarrassed to answer a second time.

"You should tape it to your body! Sixth place in the whole entire country! Wow!" She smiled as he moved on to another Tracey, the smallest girl on the stage. He pointed the microphone at her. "What about you? What did you place?"

"Twenty-third," she said, head bowed.

"What did they give you? A piece of rug?"

The audience howled. It was funny. We all laughed as he sat there smugly on his stool, winking kindly in Tracey Calore's direction, letting her know it was okay to place twenty-third. It was hilarious, all of it. Even to us, because we knew it didn't matter what he said. We wouldn't have even been there talking to him if we hadn't been winners. No matter what we'd placed, we were special. And he knew we could laugh at his jokes at our own expense. It didn't matter if he teased us to get a few laughs. We were all in collusion—he'd make fun of us, we'd walk away feeling even more like winners than if we'd taken the whole competition. At home, the girls in our elementary and junior high schools weren't competing at championships, staying in a fancy hotel, standing onstage being teased by Bill Cosby. We felt distinguished.

Upon my return to school, I didn't talk about my experience. There didn't seem to be a way to tell my classmates about it without coming across as boastful. "I went to championships and I placed thirteenth and I met Bill Cosby." They would snidely whisper that I was "conceited," the ultimate insult slung by preteen girls. I also feared that, though my thirteenth-place finish in the world of gymnastics was admirable, it seemed like nothing much to a bunch of middle-schoolers who didn't distinguish between thirteenth place in our class, the state, or the country. I kept my accomplishments to myself in school, hiding them like secrets.

My parents were more vocal in their pride. When we returned home, they boasted to their friends about their daughter being called upon by Bill Cosby, lined up onstage with the best gymnasts in the entire country. They told of my thirteenth-place finish, explaining the strenuousness of my training, the dedication required. "Her first year!" they vaunted. "Imagine!"

They floated on the cloud of my excitement, caught up in the possibilities. They weren't swayed by Traci's head injury or her coach's blatant disregard of the life-threatening implications of landing on her head from the height of a basketball net. They laughed about Barrie's father's query. My dad was pleased with his "Get her pregnant!" response; he took a "That oughta show him!" infused with "Can you believe that guy!" attitude in the retelling.

Neither of my parents ever pondered aloud the pervasive neglect exhibited on the part of the parents and coaches, at this, my very first U.S. Championships. It seemed part of the deal at this level, for most. But abuse and neglect were not required. The Seys would be different. My parents believed we were an uncommon family. We would keep our wits about us; amidst the mêlée, we would rise above.

# Chapter 12

I WAS OFFICIALLY A MEMBER OF THE 1981 U.S. National Team. And as an official member, I was invited to compete in my first international competition, the Canadian Classic in Winnipeg. For those meets attended as a national team member, a team coach was assigned by the Gymnastics Federation. A girl's personal club coach was not permitted to attend. This was a new and frightening development. I would have the chance to prove myself to national team coaches and officials. But I would be on my own, without Lolo to coddle me. She knew my foibles. She knew how I needed to warm up, how I'd feel if I had a difficult practice before a competition, how to boost my confidence if things didn't improve, how to mollify me when my self-flagellation got a little too intense. She knew when I needed a break and when I needed a push. Without the safety and indulgent encouragement I received from Lolo, I didn't know what to expect of myself. I was twelve years old, dependent on the guidance of a coach who knew how to get the best out of me.

Gary, from the Maryland MarVaTeens, was assigned as the team coach. And Mary, the choreographer I'd encountered at the California compulsory clinic, was the assistant coach. There were six girls on the squad, half of us without the benefit of a familiar coach. Traci Hinkle, the girl with the concussion, was there on her own. Though she hadn't finished at championships, she was invited to attend this meet after other girls bowed out, an indication of its lack of significance on the international circuit. Amy Appler, from Berks in Pennsylvania, was also there. She and I were acquainted from the Parkettes camp years earlier. The other three belonged to Gary or Mary. I felt like I'd been left alone in the woods to find my way home.

Still, I became friends with the gymnasts. Here competitors were also my teammates. I was no longer competing for myself. I was competing for the United States Gymnastics Team. Our goal was to place in the top six.

When we weren't practicing, we gathered in one another's rooms. We did one another's hair and pooled our team paraphernalia to trade with the girls from other countries. It was customary to bring Levi's blue jeans to trade with the Russians, USA Gymnastics pins to trade with everyone else. A collection of global pins was proof of seniority on the international scene. We also traded clothes, trying on one another's prized items. Our outfits were generally identical, but as with all adolescent girls, each sweater, each blouse, each pair of pants always seemed more desirable if it belonged to a friend. Our clothes consisted mainly of black stirrup pants and oversized V-neck sweaters worn over paisley printed blouses. It was the eighties. But somehow I looked better in Maya's and she looked better in Gigi's. Or so we thought. We curled our bangs until they were nearly singed off. We Aqua Netted them so crisp, they stood perpendicular from our foreheads. We applied makeup to one another, heavy blue eyeliner and bright purple mascara.

I didn't get a chance to do these normal girly things with the kids at home. I was relatively friendless in school as I spent most of my time at the gym. There were no after-school playdates or recreational sports teams for me. No movies on Saturday afternoons with girlfriends. After a while, the kids stopped inviting me because I always had an excuse: "I have workout" or "I have to go to the gym." "You always go there," they'd say. "Can't you miss one time?" I'd crinkle my brow in utter befuddlement. Absolutely not. It was unthinkable to miss even one day in a five-day-a-week practice schedule.

We arrived in Canada a week early to train. Mary pushed me harder than I was used to. During warm-ups, she stretched me so aggressively I thought I'd break in two. Coaches often stretched girls, bending their legs beyond what was comfortable, beyond what was painful. The goal was to enhance flexibility, stretching the muscles in the legs to allow for split leaps that extended beyond a perfect line, one leg kicked out in the front, the other behind, the hips lower than the ankles. The intent was to achieve hamstrings so loose that when a straddled handstand was performed on the beam, the legs bent in an arc, beyond 180 degrees, impossibly lithe and yielding. Lolo stretched us, but in a laid-back, comfortable way. I was naturally flexible, so she didn't find it necessary to push me in this regard. She accepted my inherent capacity without insisting that I go further.

Mary pushed me. She laid me on my back, one leg on the ground, one perpendicular to my body, pointing skyward. She managed to hold my legs in such a way that they couldn't bend, so I couldn't escape or even find relief from the pain she was inflicting. She straddled her body atop the leg on the floor, holding it steadfastly in place. Then, with the full weight of her body, she leaned on my other leg, pressing it over my head until the top of my foot was flat on the ground behind my head. She wasn't thin. And she applied her full weight onto my slight eighty-pound physique. It hurt. Tears welled in my eyes. Her Australian accent mocked me. "Is that okay?" she asked, not really wanting a reply. I squeaked in assent, trying to force a smile.

The muscles on the backs of my legs were so sore on the second day of training that I could barely run down the vault runway. But I didn't let on. I felt about Mary the way I'd felt about Janet, the University of Pennsylvania dance coach, and Patrick, the Parkettes coach I'd met at camp. I was afraid of her. Mary let her own girls have it. She screamed with every stumble, every bent leg, each minor bobble.

"Jesus, Maya, what are you, drunk?! Ten more. In a row! C'mon, c'mon!"

"Gigi, I'll send you home. Let's go. Stick ten in a row. No bobbles. No leg bends. Now!"

While she didn't muster much of a berating for girls who weren't from her club, she yelled at her own with all the spit and ire she could gather. I was terrified. I'd do exactly as I was asked, to fend off the humiliation of possibly being the first non-Mary's girl she decided to unleash her fury upon. Obedient to a fault, forever fearful of disapproval, I ran down that vault runway as if my life depended on it. Despite the aching hamstring, the severe pull she caused that would later fray into a full-fledged tear, I sprinted toward the springboard at the end of the runway as if my mother waited for me. With ice cream.

My self-doubt led me to believe these coaches had low expectations of me in this competition. I felt vulnerable and unendorsed without a major coach or club behind me. Mary's stretching techniques led me to assume my training lacked the rigor with which these well-known coaches prepared their girls. I thought that in their minds, I was not a girl to be cultivated.

They confirmed my assumption when the event order was assigned. It was generally understood that the girl who went first for her team, on any given event, got the lowest score. The judges couldn't begin by handing out big numbers. They would run out of high scores to dole out as the rotation advanced. The scores tended to get higher with each girl, whether or not the performances improved. Of course, a coach always preferred that his club girls were placed as close to the end of a rotation as possible, guaranteeing she'd be honored with the highest marks, setting her up for individual medals. Whether or not she deserved them. The coach reasoned he was protecting the team score, when really he was only protecting his own girls.

To the unfortunate first-up girl, the national team coach inevitably sold the placement as a way to "get us off to a strong start." Clap, clap. Pat on the back. But we knew better. Those of us who secured the first-up spot were sacrificial lambs. We were unprotected and unlucky, our club coaches banished from the premises by the Gymnastics Federation ("only one U.S. coach on the floor to prevent bickering and favoritism," or so the theory went). The assigned national team coaches thought we couldn't win, so we were sent ahead to feel things out, to lay the foundation for the real champs to shine.

I was placed first or second in the rotation on every event in the Canadian Classic. Lolo was not there to represent me. Gary and Mary put their girls toward the end of the rotation on all four events, drawing straws to determine which girl got the plum last-up spot. I would have been satisfied with a third-up slot on my best event, the floor exercise, giving me a chance at an individual medal. No such luck.

But I surprised them. I nailed every routine. Not a single fall. My competitiveness and mental toughness overwhelmed their girls' rigorous preparation. I didn't perform the flashiest routines, the hardest sets, but I didn't miss. Slow and steady, I eked out every routine without a major mistake. I placed on uneven bars, my worst event. And much to everyone's surprise, I snuck in to secure second place in the all-around, clinching the highest U.S. placement. I kept my head, made my routines, got the team off to a good start on each and every event, and beat all of the other U.S. girls in the process.

Because I'd missed nearly two weeks of school, the kids at home knew I'd been gone for a competition. An absence excuse was required. When I returned to class, my few school friends gathered around me, led by their queen, Rachel the dancer.

"Did you win?" the queen quipped.

How to respond? "I got the silver medal."

"But did you win?"

With a head toss, she turned on her heel, her minions following behind.

"She thinks she's so great. She didn't even win." Her followers trailed in birdlike formation, leaving me speechless and shamed.

I may not have had any close girlfriends at The Philadelphia School, but I had Angie. Though she attended public school in Willingboro, we spent the rest of our time together at the gym. And she spent many weekends at my house as well. It was lavish and privileged compared with hers. She'd sleep over, we'd giggle late into the night, talking about boys, school, gymnastics, and Michael Jackson. We filled a shoe box of newspaper clippings and magazine articles about our favorite pop star while listening to his *Off the Wall* and *Thriller* albums. We memorized the choreography of the *Thriller* music video, performing the ghoulish zombie moves showcased on MTV's most spectacular music event. My mom sat on our green corduroy couch in the living room, watching us, pleased that I finally had a friend with whom I could enjoy sleepovers and preteen girl activities.

During the summer, Lolo invited us to her vacation house at the Jersey shore for a week. My family was invited as well. I'm sure the invitation was extended to Angie's parents, but they didn't go. They both worked very hard to keep Angie's gymnastics necessities paid for. There were innumerable expenses—travel to meets, leotards, handgrips, beam shoes. Angie also had to have the right clothes in which to travel to the competitions. Her mother wouldn't have had it any other way. These things were a strain for her family. Her mother wore the same flimsy raincoat each winter so that Angie could have the right clothes.

My mom and aunt joined us at the shore. We stayed at Lolo's beach house with her grown children. We were truly part of the family. We'd wake to bagels and juice, eggs, and bacon, whipped up by Lolo. Sam, her "big-boned" son, could down three whole bagels with cream cheese and bacon before eight o'clock in the morning. My mom and I rolled our eyes and stuck out our tongues in exaggerated revulsion. We had a strong distaste for gluttony. Forbearance was revered in our house, and my mother and I nibbled our half bagels with barely a smear of cream cheese, satisfied in our obvious superiority.

After breakfast we'd all head to the beach, hot concrete pavement beneath our bare feet. We'd run all the way to avoid blistering our soles. We never thought to wear shoes during the summer. Then we'd spend the day on the sand. Angie and

I turned back handsprings and held handstands as the waves lapped against our faces. We wowed the other kids who clumsily stumbled at the water's edge, attempting awkward cartwheels for cheerleading tryouts in the fall. Gymnastics was still play for us. Even on vacation, we couldn't resist.

My dad joined us over the weekend, and we all went out on a boat for some waterskiing. Angie was afraid of the water and refused to give it a try. This apparently was her only fear. Lolo, despite being fifty years old and never having done it, gave it a go. She hopped into the water bound in her yellow life vest, donned the skis, and pulled herself up to a stand. She whooped and hollered as she flew across the choppy water.

This was the last perfect summer. Maybe that's why I remember it so clearly. After this, summers would become a haze of training and preseason preparatory competitions. But in the summer of 1982, I was still a kid. I trained seriously, but there was still room for ice cream, bodysurfing, and saltwater taffy on the boardwalk, for lazy days and late nights playing Monopoly.

I was happy.

My other close friend in the gym was Michelle Krupa, a brash city girl; she was an oddity in the pristine, little-girl-cute world of gymnastics. She was a senior in high school, five years older than me, eons in adolescent terms. Born and raised in Fishtown, a working-class neighborhood in Philadelphia, Michelle sometimes stayed the night at my house on Fridays. She'd drive me home from practice in her rusted-out Camaro, and we'd spend the evening watching television and eating popcorn before waking early to go to Saturday workout. Why this eighteen-year-old, bleached blond/dark roots, tough-talking Philly girl wanted to spend her Friday nights with me puzzled my parents.

The other girls her age—Suzie and Donna—had already

quit. And their suburban sensibilities hadn't included Michelle. Even if they'd still been in the gym, they would not have included her in their weekends. She would have been an embarrassment to bring to their idyllic, provincial high school dances with her crude city talk and trashy looks. Though our family also resided in a bedroom community in suburban New Jersey, my father worked in Philadelphia and my brother and I went to school there. We considered ourselves appropriately metropolitan and open-minded. To me, hanging out with Michelle seemed perfectly normal. Most notably, despite our age difference, we felt a kinship in our second-best status. Though Suzie was no longer practicing, her ghost was Michelle's rival, as Angie in the flesh was mine.

The gym kids were always drawn to our house. My parents were "cool." They weren't separated or into second marriages, they didn't mind our cursing—in fact my mom cursed quite a bit herself ("Where are my fucking car keys?!")—and of course, we had nice things. We were early cable subscribers, one of the first families to get a VCR. My dad made obstacle courses in the backyard with old mattresses, tires, and ropes. He'd time my brother, Michelle, and me as we muddled through the course. I think my stable, supportive, financially secure family life gave Michelle a sense of calm she never experienced in her own cramped, loud North Philly residence. She simply enjoyed being at our house.

One night, Michelle and I decided to make chocolate chip cookies for our evening of television watching. As we whipped up the ingredients, my mom sat at the kitchen table gabbing with us. While we were waiting for the cookies to bake, the conversation turned to Gary Goodson. He had no fondness for either of us. We both operated by forcible will rather than scientific exactitude. We agreed, he was a jackass. We began laughing uncontrollably. It was such a relief to make fun of this man who tormented us. Her laughing escalated, tears rolled down her face. I looked down and there was a puddle beneath her cane chair. Michelle had peed on the floor. Tears of hysteria shook our bodies. We were united in our hatred of this egomaniac, this self-appointed king of coaches who delighted in disparaging us. Finally, we could laugh about it.

Michelle and Angie were my closest friends. While socio-economic disparities would have normally prevented us from meeting and becoming pals, gymnastics brought us together. Although Michelle would be heading to college soon, hopefully on a gymnastics scholarship, our age difference was not a barrier to friendship; rather, it prevented us from being direct competitors, enabling companionship unhindered by antagonism.

Despite the intimate friendship I shared with Angie outside the gym, my envy inside the gym's walls persisted. In every national competition she consistently placed higher than me by at least three places. She had her feet firmly planted in the top ten, while I lingered outside it, in the low teens. Because she had a higher rank on the national team, she was picked for a far more prestigious assignment for her first international competition.

One inauspicious evening practice, a call came into the gym for Lolo. A federation official told her that one of the senior girls invited to attend the Riga Cup in Latvia had an injury. Could Angie attend? The meet was just a week away.

Lolo told Angie, who of course was thrilled. It was an honor. This was an important competition. All the best in the world would be there—the Romanians, the Russians, the Hungarians. Immediately I became sullen and bitter. This was clearly an indication that she was *much* better than me. While I knew she was a little better, I'd fooled myself into believing we were pretty equal. I was only a few places behind in the national ranking, after all. And she had been training more seriously than I had for a longer time. Surely, it was just a matter of time before I caught up and then surpassed her. But this. It took the wind out of me, like a blow to the chest. Tears blurred my vision as I tried to continue with my balance beam practice. I tried to keep my welling anger and resentment to myself. Lolo could see I was seething. I hadn't even given Angie a congratulatory hug. Lolo called me over, put an arm around me, soothed my bruised ego but at the same time encouraged me to be a gracious young lady, a graceful competitor. A friend. I wanted no part of that.

"My parents wouldn't let me go there anyway. It's dangerous," I spat, so Angie could hear me. In one statement I'd hissed as many mean sentiments as were possible. My parents cared about me more than hers did. It wasn't really an honor to be invited to this competition in such an unpredictable part of the world. But I was hurt. I couldn't help myself. Lolo sent me home. She kicked me out to prevent me from saying any more insulting things to Angie, my supposed best friend, to prevent me from injuring myself (I was too upset to safely finish my practice), and to punish me for my mean-spiritedness. There was nothing worse than missing practice. Especially now, when it was clear I had a lot of work to do if I was going to catch up to Angie. To eventually beat her.

I went home as instructed, too stubborn to apologize, too wounded to put it so quickly behind me. The game was on. My competitive ire was invoked. I would triumph over Angie. I would leave this favorite girl, this talented athlete, my best friend, in the dust. She wasn't going to top me. No way.

**Chapter 13**  In 1982 MY GOAL WAS TO BREAK into the top ten. Qualifying for USA Championships was not an issue. I'd already done it once; I was a veteran. Making it into the most celebrated competition in the United States no longer seemed like something praiseworthy. It was just a required step in my new mission.

Despite my nonchalance about qualifying, this year seemed a much bigger deal somehow. The junior and senior elites would compete in the same arena in Salt Lake City. When Angie and I practiced at the site in the days before the meet, all of my idols were there: Tracee Talavera, Lisa Zeis, Julianne McNamara, Kelly Garrison. They were all in the same meet that I was in. There would be television cameras there to capture the seniors' competition for Saturday-afternoon live sports programming. These senior girls were the ones who would comprise the Olympic Team in two years if they could keep it together, maintain their focus, prevent their bodies from falling apart. I was awed. These were the girls pictured on posters hanging in my room.

When we worked out in the arena, I experienced a level of nervousness that was new to me. It all seemed more weighty and important, like I'd finally "made it" and my future career in gymnastics hinged on this particular meet. My hands shook. I couldn't speak. There was a knot in my throat the size of a tennis ball. And it showed. I struggled all week on balance beam. For the life of me, I couldn't stay on that plank. My side aerial, a cartwheel with no hands, gave me the most problems. Not a particularly difficult trick, it gave me a C-rated skill needed to meet the minimal requirements. But I hadn't made one all week. Each time, I fell to the ground. The more I labored, the more times I hurriedly threw my body into the aerial, the less control I had. My frustration mounted. And as it did, my performance worsened. I had no sense of my center of gravity. I was wavering up on that four-foot-high girder, wishing, hoping I could find the glue that would keep me stuck. In the end, having thrown and failed nearly one hundred aerials during the course of the week, Lolo asked me if I'd like to take it out of my routine for the competition. She left the decision to me, and I decided it would be best to remove the treacherous skill. I reasoned the deduction for not meeting the requirements would be less than for the fall.

Angie, of course, struggled with nothing that week. Clear-headed and lighthearted, she approached the competition without fear. She always went into these meets with an "Oh well" attitude. She felt as if she was lucky to be there and whatever the outcome, it was merely icing on the proverbial cake. She enjoyed herself a lot more than I did. My gut twisted in angst as I calculated scores that would allow me to top her in the rankings.

Traci Hinkle, fully healed from her head injury in Reno, was there with a new team, the Parkettes. She'd left her coach, whom I now knew as Bruce, after the Reno incident. Her new coaches, the Strausses, weren't rumored to be much kinder, but they hid their missteps more skillfully and had a cadre of girls ranked in the top ten already. Traci's former teammate Heather was there with Bruce, the man known by now to be a loose cannon. Once again, he made a scandalous scene one day in practice, screaming foul epithets ("Stupid little bitch!") and slapping the backs of Heather's legs when she couldn't stay on the bars. He threatened not to coach her during the meet and held true to his word. During the competition he was nowhere to be found. She went through it alone, setting her own bars at the proper distance and pliancy, placing her own vault board the preferred distance from the horse. Psyching herself up before each event. Patting herself on the back after each routine. For a girl of thirteen, she was remarkably calm and self-assured in the face of being abandoned by the adult who was supposed to provide encouragement and keep her safe.

Heather's parents watched her go about the competition alone. They cheered from the stands, their Texas twang heard above the din, while shrugging off Bruce's behavior as part of the deal. They assumed his disciplinary tactics were essential to get the best out of their daughter. His immature, tyrannical outburst would have been averted if she'd performed better, made fewer mistakes, they reasoned. She'd brought it on with her imperfection.

My mom and dad, who sat with Heather's parents during the meet, were horrified at their complacency. They expected a coach to be along the lines of a Lolo—a kind, considerate teacher, not a crazed, self-indulgent child abuser. They didn't assume Bruce's behavior was endemic to the best coaches in the sport. They felt protected in their selection of Lolo and in the knowledge that they would never tolerate such abuses heaped upon their daughter. They assumed Heather's parents' reaction had something to do with their tough-talking Texan roots and that worldly, sophisticated Jews from the Philadelphia area would never put up with this kind of thing. They presumed they would know if it was happening because it would be public, like this. They thought I would reject such treatment, stand up for myself, flee. I was a sensible, strong-willed girl, and the Seys were a close-knit family. This could never happen to us. Lolo's kindness in the face of my difficulties in practice all week was proof.

Taking out the side aerial proved judicious. I stayed on the beam during the meet. Lolo had a hug for me after my dismount, proud that I was able to overcome my frustration and land a respectable score in the high 8s. This cautious approach kept me happy in the short term and, ultimately, shaped my approach to competition. Don't fall. Get through the routines. Don't take any chances. While high 8s may sound low compared with the perfect 10s celebrated in the Olympics, an all-around score consisting of high 8s and low 9s was enough to place a junior in the top twelve, the national team cutoff. I managed twelfth place this time, topping my performance from the prior year by one slot but missing my goal.

Disappointed that I was unable to take my place with Angie in that illusory top squad (she was ninth), I accepted my seeding with humility. There were no tears or nasty asides directed at Angie. But I wondered: Will Lolo get me there? Traci had left her coach less than a year ago and scooted up the rankings to the coveted top ten in this competition. Her new coaches were rumored to be nasty, but they got her where I wanted to be. I was impatient. Would I need to move on to other coaches, more rigorous methods at a more highly recognized gym, to get my top-ten ranking? Despite Lolo's unconditional love and careful guidance and the fact that she always had my best interest as a young girl close to her heart, I thought to myself, *I don't want someone who considers me as a person. I want someone who can make me a winner.* That was all I cared about. How would I break top ten. Then top six. It was imperative to do so as a junior so that I'd be well positioned by the time I turned fifteen. So that once I competed as a senior I would be widely recognized as one of the best. So that I would be a shoo-in for a top-six ranking in the fifteen-and-over category, an obvious choice to send to the World Championships and the Olympics.

I constantly moved the goal line. Nothing I achieved was ever sufficient. I never took a moment to bask in the glory, to appreciate my accomplishments. It was always, "How do I get to the next level?" Thirteen years old, ranked twelfth in the country, and I was filled with self-loathing. Two spots shy of my goal just wasn't good enough. I could do more.

But I had a looming sense of the very narrow window of opportunity afforded me in gymnastics. Mortality hovered persistently. Time was of the essence. Each passing year represented the narrowing of the window, the tightening of the vise. Even the best gymnasts didn't usually compete beyond age eighteen. Some girls stuck it out until their twenties, but they were few and far between. And somehow, these competitors, the "old ones," young women still playing with little girls, seemed a little pathetic. They were afraid to leave the safety net, the known success of gymnastics. They were afraid to become adults.

And all of us, even those who competed into adulthood, would have to find second careers once we retired. These second-choice career options were tainted with the dim, near-death patina of aging retirees working at Wal-Mart to fill the time and supplement their Social Security checks. Not so for baseball and basketball players, golfers, football stars. The best made lifelong careers out of their athletic prowess. For the gymnast, it was all over, abruptly, before college even started. We were ready for retirement when most kids were moving out on their own, ready to take on the world.

I knew I had to achieve very quickly in order to beat the menacing development of my own body, to shine with undeniable brightness in my adolescent career, before giving it all up for the old-age home. I had to break in to the top six before puberty and curves and weight made it nearly impossible for me to fly through the air, attempting flips meant for younger, lighter girls.

So, the slow crawl from thirteenth to twelfth, a one-slot improvement from one year to the next, would never be good enough. I had to jump ahead more radically, improve my placement at a much more aggressive rate. I had an impending sense of the day my "past due" status would be staring me in the face. Quietly, I contemplated my next move.

# Chapter 14

DESPITE MY DISAPPOINTMENT after 1982 championships, I was honored with invitations to compete in a number of international and national meets for the U.S. team. I seized these opportunities to prove myself as a virtuous national team member. Angie was out of the picture for the time being, her bunions inflicting discomfort not worth fighting through. She took a year's break from competition, fastening her feet into contraptions intended to reduce the size of the nodules. Her absence from practice made me the star, mitigating my desire to find another club immediately. As the best girl in the gym training for international meets, I was satisfied for the time being.

Though gymnastics manufactured obstacles for me—a pulled hamstring that was sore and growing into a tear, an ankle perpetually swollen from short landings—I refused to let them interfere with my plans. This was the year that I would prove that *I* was the worthy girl from Will-Moor.

Two weeks before I was set to leave for Tokyo to represent

the United States in competition, I fainted in the shower, weak with fever. By the next morning, the chicken pox had exploded into pustules on my face, chest, and back. Now it was everyday life, not gymnastics-inflicted injury, that I would have to barrel through. Despite the fact that I was unable to practice in the days leading up to the competition, I refused to forfeit my spot. I'd healed beyond contagion in time to board the plane to Japan. My face was scabby with healing pox, but crusty blisters weren't going to keep me from flying halfway around the world to compete for my country. And any meet without Angie afforded me the opportunity to shine. To emerge from the shadows. In my mind, she was the only one who blocked my light. Other girls could beat me, but it only needled when Angie did. I wouldn't have missed this meet for anything.

I did all right. No medals, but no falls either. It was a checkmark on my personal report card—I traveled as far as Angie competing for the national team.

The short trip to Japan—four days in total—was monumental. I traveled with one other girl and her coach, chosen by the federation to accompany us. My parents didn't chaperone. Lolo stayed home with Angie. Armed with calamine lotion and chutzpah, I entered the world of truly international competition. My one prior experience, Canada, hardly counted; I hadn't even left the continent. In Tokyo, I fought the jet lag that accompanied a thirteen-hour time change and twenty-hour plane ride and competed honorably. I visited Osaka Castle, rode the bullet train to catch a view of Mount Fuji, and waded through the markets of downtown Tokyo to try the sushi and dried fish. I bought Sony Walkmen and Asics Tiger sneakers for my brother and me. And I returned home triumphant and transformed, fully comfortable in my role as a worldly wise junior national team member and suitably inspired to climb the ranks.

Later that year, I attended the National Sports Festival, a meet that split male and female U.S. hopefuls into teams of green, yellow, red, and blue to compete as "countries" against one another for a championship cup. From around the country, we descended on the Colorado Springs Olympic Training Center. We were assigned austere rooms with cots and scratchy blankets. It was like summer camp, except girls and boys boarded together in one dormitory.

Most of the girls were under fifteen, whereas the boys were college-aged. Comparably developed male gymnasts were always five or more years older than their female counterparts, their version of the sport requiring strength that only came with full physical maturity. We girls giggled late into the night, talking about all the cute college boys. We snuck out to the convenience mart, darting across the freeway to buy candy and soda. We played Ping-Pong and air hockey in the recreation center, hoping to get a turn against Mitch, the height of flirtation for a group of thirteen-year-olds enamored with college freshmen. The slightly older and more developed girls went beyond flirting. It was rumored that one of the more physically mature girls had had sex with one of the guys. But I was shy. I tried not to look when Chris from Nebraska tried to get my attention in the cafeteria. This was the sleep-away camp I'd never attended.

For the competition, the least exciting part of this affair, I was assigned to the blue team. Again, I was there without Angie. She was still on the injured list, her malformed feet flared, red with pain. I relaxed when she wasn't there. Because she was still my closest friend, when we traveled together we were inseparable. It became unavoidable that I was the big, slow girl compared with her. When she wasn't there, suddenly there was no comparison. I was just Jen, not big, not fat, not soft, not second to anyone.

During practice the day before the competition, a boy on

the red team was swinging on high bar. He was building up speed, showing off a bit for a female red teammate. As he cranked his swing and then released, he soared over the metal rod that served as the high bar. But when he reached for the bar, his fingertips grazed it, unable to fully grasp. The bar twanged loudly with the force of his miss. He crashed into the mat, hands before face, sending chalk dust flying. When he didn't get up, the trainer rushed to his aid to find blood pooling on the mat beneath his cheek. Upon impact, his neck crashed down onto his handgrip, the buckle cutting into his throat. He was rushed to the hospital, woozy from blood loss, lucky to have missed the jugular vein.

Again, misfortune struck the men during the competition when another young man suffered a disastrous fall. With the full speed of a run behind him, his feet slipped from the vault board and he collided with the horse, gut first. On the men's vault, the horse was aligned with the runway, forming one straight line, the force of his crash concentrated by the narrow point of contact. (For women at the time, the horse was perpendicular to the runway, forming a T shape, diffusing a crash of this sort.) He was knocked unconscious and rushed to the hospital.

The true danger of the sport was brought home to me. Throwing the body through the air, performing ill-advised flips and twists off of unforgiving poles and beams, were things to be taken seriously. While I knew danger threatened with every new trick thrown, I had never witnessed bloody, devastating injuries up close. The nagging muscle pulls, the sore wrists and ankles, were nothing compared with the near-catastrophic falls that prowled the gym floor, waiting to lead an unsuspecting gymnast to her demise.

In 1983 I suffered my first significant injury. It was not of the catastrophic variety, rather the type born from overuse. My torn hamstring began as an irritating pull, sustained in the Canadian Classic, but soon grew into a debilitating obstacle. It is a common affliction among young, growing gymnasts, given the strain put on the muscles. The fact that the hamstring must behave strongly and flexibly at the same moment creates undue strain. A muscle is generally asked to do one thing at a time—hold weight (requiring strength), bend, or flex (requiring pliancy). But, simple gymnastics skills such as front aerials—a no-handed front walkover—demand that the leg is stretched while the muscle is taut and straining. My hamstring tore at the base, where it connected to the buttocks. It was weakened considerably, often giving out on me while I ran toward the vault or leapt on the beam.

Doctors didn't diagnose it. There was no bruising. No visible signs of tearing. No dangling muscle beneath the skin. Nothing showed on an X-ray. Other than pain, I was fine. I refused to miss a meet. Without a firm diagnosis, there was no reason to.

I went to 1983 U.S. Championships in Chicago, performing terribly, the pain and weakness in my leg too much to bear. Floor exercise, usually a strong event for me, was disastrous. I suffered two major falls, the result of a slow approach and compromised takeoff. This was a lost season, nothing accomplished in my final year as a junior gymnast. I had fallen in the ranks, rather than ascending as planned, setting myself up for a difficult first year out as a senior. While I was crying at the end of the competition, Tracee Talavera, a 1980 Olympic Team member and an idol of mine, put an arm around me. She eyed the ice pack bandaged to my hamstring.

"You're hurt," she said. I nodded. "It's okay, Jen. Your beam looked good. You'll do better next time."

How did she know my name? I was honored. She had had

a rough meet as well, placing in the low 20s. Coaches were talking of a failed comeback. She had been the young hotshot just a few years earlier, and already she was considered over the hill, needing to make a *comeback* if she was going to qualify for the Olympics in 1984. Yet she held her head high, gave me a pat on the back. She didn't cry. She was proud, a graceful competitor, the exception to the rule in a sport rampant with childish behavior on the part of the athletes and coaches alike. I determined at that moment that I, too, would smile, hold my head high. Sitting with her, I made the choice to set an example as an adult among children. I would compete with poise and finish with character, whether things went my way or not.

After the disappointment of the 1983 USA Championships, I started high school, an even more harrowing experience. I was inordinately nervous about attending public school in Haddonfield. I was used to my urban liberal private school in Philadelphia, where I enjoyed small classes, learning at my own pace, and a test-less environment. Though I had inflicted pressure upon myself, I had faced almost none of the normal externally applied academic or peer pressures of junior high. But my parents sent me to the public high school in our town to introduce a bit of normalcy into my life. The kids there had all gone to school together since first grade. They had forged lifelong friendships. I was an outsider.

While high school proved to be an adjustment—the cavernous hallways; the rigid classrooms where we all learned together at the same crawling pace, no matter how bored some of us were; the cliques of popular girls who made fun of scrawny, immature nerds—tests, the thing I most feared, turned out to be my friend. I posted consistent A's without much effort. The good grades didn't mean much to me because they were so easy to achieve, hardly worth self-congratulation. They also didn't do much for my popularity. Straight A's were a surefire way to cement my position as a strange and unwanted interloper.

I had one friend at Haddonfield High. Janine Schissler. The picture-perfect nerd, she wore glasses, played on the tennis team, and aspired to Harvard. Though she'd attended Haddonfield public schools her entire life, it seemed she hadn't really made any friends. She sat beside me in homeroom and adopted me on the very first day of school. I was grateful. At least it was someone to walk to class with, to borrow notes from if I missed classes for a competition or an early workout. We had all of our classes together: honors geometry, chemistry, and English.

Janine introduced me to my first boyfriend, Jimmy Groling. They were acquainted from the tennis team. He was also nerdy—red-haired, freckled, gangly—but he wafted between the popular kids and the brainy ones. Being the class clown made him acceptable in most circles. And he liked me enough to ask me on a date. We went to the movies on a Saturday afternoon. He paid for the PG film, and then we snuck into the R-rated *Purple Rain,* starring pop star Prince. Nabbed by the usher, despite sinking deep into our seats to avoid detection, we were escorted out of the theater. This made the date more memorable and bond-worthy than if we had sat through the sex scenes between Prince and Apollonia, certainly the reason he had wanted to see the film in the first place. While I'm sure he was anxious to gauge my response to the lasciviousness in the movie, thus benchmarking my receptivity to this kind of activity, he ultimately made more progress in softening my defenses when we had to flee the theater in fits of laughter.

Our second date was a school dance. There, on the dance floor, which doubled as the gymnasium's basketball court during school hours, he kissed me. For the very first time, a boy kissed me. It was relatively unmoving. His tongue was pointy and dry. But we stuck to it for at least an hour. When I got home, I was giddy. I couldn't sleep. I pulled the covers up to my chin and replayed the kissing over and over in my head. The mechanical feel of it. The hard jabbing of his darty tongue. My heart racing despite the lack of passion. Over and over, the thought floated in my head: Finally, I'm normal.

We proceeded to date for a few months. I went to his tennis matches on the weekends. I was teased at school, the thought being that my gymnastic ability had some bearing on my sexual prowess. I wasn't sure what Jimmy had said to instigate that, but I didn't mind. He had popular friends who now knew my name. I was in. I would not be made fun of anymore—called "baby" or "dork" or "dyke," as some of the girls in the locker room whispered, because I excelled on the chin-up bar and snuck peeks at the other girls, full-breasted, as they changed into their gym clothes. (I hadn't seen teenagers with such developed figures; friends in the gym were as straight up and down as I was.) Jimmy and I went to more dances, made out. The public displays helped my reputation. I wasn't a complete loser anymore.

Sometimes Jimmy invited me to his house, where we hung out in the basement under the guise of watching TV or playing Ping-Pong. But he'd spend most of the time trying to get me to sit next to him on the couch while I lingered clear across the room, perched on a weight-lifting bench. I stood my ground, maintaining distance, refusing to kiss him in the basement, afraid where it might lead and how I'd be expected to comply. I never overtly refused; I just kept away from the couch, close to the safety of the weight-lifting machines. He never insisted I come sit next to him. He was sweet. He hoped, but never demanded, to get a hand under my shirt. He would have found a chest as flat and bare as his own. But he wouldn't have cared. Despite my lack of womanliness, he could've bragged to his friends that he'd felt up the gymnast. This alone wouldn't have bothered me. I wasn't afraid of having a reputation as unchaste (this would have just made me closer to average amongst my libidinous classmates); I was afraid of sex or anything close to it.

Once I'd been the object of Jimmy's longing, I realized I didn't feel the need to be desired. I didn't crave sexual attention like many girls my age. I wanted only to be admired, to be an accomplished champion. And I had a limited window of opportunity to do so. The sex stuff could come later. In fact, I felt shamed when desirous attention was cast my way. That was something reserved for women, and I considered myself a girl. While others my age were striving to appear older than their years, to drink and smoke and engage in heavy petting, I ached to remain a little girl. Women were rarely seen on the competitive floor and certainly never won medals that allowed them to climb the podium. Only little girls won in gymnastics.

Coldheartedly, I broke up with Jimmy over the phone, a respectable three months after that first kiss. He was devastated. I didn't understand his protestations. "Please," he begged, "I won't pressure you. We don't have to do anything you don't want to do. We don't even have to actually go anywhere. Just be my girlfriend." I was dumbfounded. I thought he'd just consent with an "Okay, see you at school." I thought he was playacting this whole thing with me. But he was actually pleading. He was desperate.

While I understood the desire to appear normal, I didn't want to actually *be* normal. Jimmy was the perfect foil—an actual male to fulfill the promise of "boyfriend." But he was still a boy, his sexual attentions mediated by his unimposing physicality. He was skinny and nonthreatening, so I used him to get my first kiss. I'd never felt any emotional attachment. But his desire was to *be* normal, to have a girlfriend. He wanted to hold hands in the halls at school, steal a kiss between classes, slide a hand up under my shirt. And he may have actually liked me, a little bit, as drawn to my awkwardness as I was to his. So he pleaded. He cried. Unsympathetic, I bluntly explained that I just wasn't ready for a real relationship. I told him I wasn't like other high school kids. I preferred to be with my family, playing board games or going to the movies on Friday nights, going to bed early to rest up for the coming week. "Please, don't," he begged.

"I just don't want a boyfriend." I hung up the phone, liberated. There would be no more basement sessions, no more dry kisses, no more weaseling out of Friday-night keg parties at So-and-So's house. Janine told me that Jimmy was spotted recklessly drunk, the very night I'd broken up with him. He didn't drink, as far as I knew. And that purported drunken night hadn't even been accomplished at a party where drunkenness was the goal. He'd done it on his own. Because he was broken up about me. I felt honored. I chalked it up as experience.

# Chapter 15

In 1984, I missed the entire competition season. My first year as a senior gymnast, I skipped the elite qualifying zone meet due to the pain caused by my hamstring injury. Though I had been an elite as a junior, the jump in age category required that I requalify. I couldn't bear the thought of an embarrassing performance like the one I'd logged in Chicago championships the prior year. I resolved to forgo an almost certainly disappointing showing to allow myself to heal. Angie sat out the year as well, succumbing to the pain of sore feet once again. I took solace in knowing that she wouldn't pull ahead of me any more than she already was. She was my personal unit of measure, the nearest yardstick that I sized myself up against. There were others who were better, who would provide more worthy and far-reaching inspiration, but like siblings who only measure their accomplishments against each other's, Angie provided all the motivation I needed.

The fact that it was an Olympic year was a distraction from

my personal setback. Many of the 1980 Olympic Team members continued through to 1984 to realize their goal of competing in the Games. Injured or not, there had been no chance for me to qualify. I hadn't achieved the requisite skill, experience, or notoriety. I just wasn't good enough yet.

I certainly couldn't compare to the new darling of U.S. gymnastics, Mary Lou Retton. I knew Mary Lou from the days of the Class One regionals. She was from Fairmont, West Virginia, all power and dynamism. Back in 1979, clad in a drab yellow-and-brown leotard, she performed skills none of the other Class Ones could have fathomed, including double backs on floor and handspring front vaults in the pike position. Back then, she had trouble containing her power and she often fell, overshooting with an extra quarter or half rotation. Built squat and low to the ground, she had an audacity that more than made up for what she lacked in grace and poise.

Bela Karolyi, Nadia's former coach, was now stationed in Houston. He had seen Mary Lou's potential and recruited her in 1982, effectively harnessing her power. He took her natural skills and emphasized them beyond the U.S. gymnastics scene's collective imagination. Her double layout on floor (two somersaults in the air, the body in a fully stretched and straight position) appeared effortless. No other U.S. gymnast came close to performing anything this mind-blowing. Her layout full Tsukahara on vault was executed to 10.0 flawlessness each and every time. Bela even leveraged her powerful athletic jumping ability into her bar routine by creating the "Retton Flip," a front somersault performed by springing from the low bar to the high, landing in a perched seated position on the upper bar. He and his wife, Marta, had also sufficiently polished her connecting dance moves on floor and her ability to stay on the balance beam to make her lack of grace a nonissue.

Mary Lou won the 1984 Olympic Trials, making her the

obvious front-runner for the United States going into the Los Angeles–hosted Games. It had been widely assumed that the Soviets would boycott, retaliating against the U.S.-led boycott of the Moscow Games. In May the USSR officially announced that they would not attend, citing myriad political reasons, including threats to their athletes and officials. The Soviets had shot down a Korean airliner on September 1, 1983, provoking reactions by the United States, the most significant being the formation of the Ban the Soviets Coalition. While the body was unimportant in and of itself, it provided something concrete that the Soviets could point to as evidence of the United States' hostility. Ultimately, thirteen Soviet allies joined the boycott. The only Soviet-bloc country that attended the Games was Romania. Despite the intervening politics, 140 nations attended, including China, returning after a thirty-two-year absence.

Mary Lou engaged in a head-to-head battle with the Romanian star Ecaterina Szabó. It was also a symbolic battle for Bela, who needed to prove that his reputation for training champions was attributable to his own coaching abilities, not the Romanian way of life. The patriotic U.S. audience was delighted by the intense rivalry that mirrored political tensions of the day. Though Mary Lou trailed Ecaterina after her first two events—bars and beam, her weakest—she pulled ahead with two perfect 10s on floor and vault, winning the all-around title by a half tenth of a point. Though Mary Lou's win was widely debated as undeserved—given that the Russians were not present—she was the incontrovertible "it" girl of the Games; she secured *Sports Illustrated*'s "Sportswoman of the Year" title and became the first woman athlete to appear on the Wheaties box, the commercial financial prize of the day.

U.S. women's gymnastics finally had a star worth boasting about to the world. I petulantly dismissed her performance as not win-worthy "if the Russians had been there." My lack of enthusiasm was a childish defense; I felt discouraged. My style of gymnastics was the opposite of Mary Lou's. I was sure the trend toward undiluted power and athleticism that she invoked would work against me in the coming years.

But her celebrity and dominance enticed me. With my hamstring almost healed, I begged my mom to let me attend Karolyi's camp. I was at yet another inflection point in my career: I'd missed my critical first year out as a senior, and I had no national ranking. The Olympic Team would surely retire to make way for a new crop of girls. I thought if I could impress Bela, current master and impresario, my ascendancy would be guaranteed.

I told Lolo I was off to camp in Houston. She didn't worry. She figured if I was going to move on to pursue my career at another gym, then that would be what was best for me. With her blessing, I enrolled like any other girl. There was no special registration for former national team members. I was mixed in with competitive novices. I stayed with a family friend, though I was never at her house. Workouts lasted most of the day, about eight hours. Bela himself was nowhere to be found during the camp sessions, but I wasn't swayed. I was sure that his minion coaches reported back about the most talented girls after tossing us through tricks we'd never attempted. I assumed they were gauging our bravery, our willingness to try anything. They had no qualms about our qualification to be trying these reckless moves like double layouts and full-in backouts (a double back with a full twist on the first somersault). If a gymnast landed on her head, broke a bone, tore a ligament, so what? These coaches were testing our mettle as well as our talent.

While I demonstrated first-rate daring, my athletic prowess was dubious. I tried everything, but I crashed and burned consistently. I repeatedly landed on my head in the foam pit—a deep cement hole in the ground filled with two-foot-square foam pieces. Over and over again, neck-crunching head landings didn't dissuade me. *Crash. Crunch.* I just bounced up and tried again. My fear was once again suppressed in the name of gleaning approval and avoiding reproach.

None of the coaches were impressed with my tenacity. My suspect athleticism trumped my work ethic, in their minds. If I had made an impression, I would have been asked to join the team immediately. I watched the team girls practice on the other side of the gym, longing to be invited to enroll. Despite the fact that the coaches hurled absurd insults at these girls ("You look like a scrawny chicken!" and "You're a fat pig!), I ached to be good enough to be a part of this team. It was a sure thing. If I practiced at Karolyi's, did everything that was asked of me, I would succeed. But they didn't want me.

Ultimately, none of the girls in my camp session were tapped to join. The standards at Karolyi's were impossibly high. Bela only wanted to train girls assured to have the makings of champions. At fifteen, I was already old. And I had no ranking or standout physical capability to set me apart. "Champion" was not stamped on my future. But I wasn't ready to give up.

"How was it?" my mom asked on the ride home from the airport.

"It's not for me."

"Do you want to go back to Will-Moor?" she asked.

"For now." I was resigned to proving myself in an upcoming competition, then reconsidering my options. Something closer to home, perhaps.

Finally, at the end of 1984, I realized a full hamstring recovery. It took nearly a year and a half for this irksome and frustrating injury to heal. As a means of easing back into competition, I led my team in the Garden State Classic, an invitational meet. Invitational meets (the host team invited other clubs to their home turf to vie for a team title) were often used by coaches as rehearsals for the more important national competitions. This meet, hosted by my team, was so late in the competition season that it actually rounded the corner into preparation for the 1985 season. While ostensibly presented as a team meet, the most prestigious medals were given for individual performances.

I was intent on making an impression. I trained harder than I ever had. I insisted on making five routines on each event, each practice. This wasn't Lolo's usual approach. She was much more fluid—if I was having a bad day, I could usually just skip an event that was giving me trouble. I knew I had to be harder on myself.

I also lost weight, something I'd never really considered actively pursuing before. The combination of harder practices and a heightened sensitivity to my own self-perceived chubbiness drove me to diet. Gary Goodson assigning me the nickname Dough Girl when I was twelve years old finally helped me recognize the necessary fact that I was just too fat. His words stuck with me, and now, at fifteen, I knew that I did not have the required lean, sinewy appearance of a champion. In making my foray into the senior ranks, I would have to correct this situation. For months I ate nothing but yogurt and apples. The Will-Moor coaches didn't encourage attention to weight, so I had to sneak up to Lolo's office each day to dust off the scale and check my status. As far as I could tell, this scale had never been used by anyone at Will-Moor. There was no weight chart where I could pencil in my progress, so I had to keep track in my head. I lost five pounds, not an alarming amount, but enough to allow the muscles to emerge in my legs. No longer puffy and ill defined, my legs now appeared strong and powerful. Not soft with baby fat or bulky with Mary Lou weight-lifter-style muscles. I was thin and strong, elegant as a dancer. For the first time, I thought I looked like a *real* gymnast.

Angie wound up not competing in the meet, refusing to join me in the comeback process. She had been struggling in practice, still using the excuse of aching bunions. She sat for hours on the sidelines during workouts, feet bound in a torture vise intended to reduce the size and tenderness of the inflamed, bony lumps. Though the pain limited her, I think she also feared losing to me. It would be a close competition between us for the first time. If she didn't compete, she wouldn't have to relinquish her superiority. She would be "letting me win" as she sat in the stands, toes pulled in all directions. A kindly service for a gymnast in need of a confidence boost. She couldn't fail if she didn't try. It would be easier to maintain the illusion of preeminence if she didn't show up to compete.

I dominated the meet. Not only did I win the all-around, I won every individual event as well. I had never won a competition before, and this time I collected five gold medals. I was as close to perfect as I could've imagined. I nailed every routine, scoring mid-9s on each event. Everyone talked about how I'd improved. "You look like a Russian," one of the young Parkette gymnasts remarked. This was the supreme compliment; the Russians were known to be the leanest—in addition to the best—competitors in the world. Coaches and judges congratulated me on my performance and my appearance. My confidence soared.

The time had come to make a choice. Though I'd handily taken the New Jersey competition, I had no national visibility. I was a senior gymnast. In 1985, a new pre-Olympic four-year cycle would be kicked off. It would be critical for me to finally break in to the top ten, if I intended to qualify for the World

Championships and then secure an Olympic Team spot in 1988. I revisited the issue with my parents. We determined that there were two gyms other than Karolyi's worth considering at the time: Parkettes in Allentown, Pennsylvania, and SCATS in Huntington Beach, California. It felt like treason to even consider switching. Lolo had been so good to me. But I knew she would understand that my priorities had changed. I found it easy to cast aside our bond, as well as my enjoyment of daily practices, because I could glimpse what winning might feel like.

My life had utter singularity of purpose. I exclusively identified myself as a gymnast. *I was a gymnast.* That was it. It was a lot. More than most kids, I thought. Most kids dallied. They passed time in school, tarried at some sport or other. They waited until they were old enough to leave home and go to college to define themselves on their own terms. I had such an unusually clear (and narrow) definition of myself. I knew myself in a way that most can only hope to get close to. Everything led to my being a gymnast. Everything receded from it. It was a clear and knowable vanishing point. Choices were uncomplicated. I simply chose the route that would allow me to become the best gymnast. *I was a gymnast.*

# Chapter 16

"LET'S TRY PARKETTES," I OFFERED one day on the way home from practice in the winter of 1984.

"Okay," my mom said, nodding with relief. Parkettes was driving distance from our house—two hours each way—a feasible though monotonous commute. I wouldn't even have to move away from home if I didn't want to. My dad offered to buy a van so that I could study comfortably while my mom drove me there and back each day. This could work, we agreed.

My mom and I went to Allentown to meet the Strausses, the Parkette founders and head coaches. Of course I'd seen them before at meets, and I was acquainted with most of the girls on the team. Still, I was nervous. I gnawed on my mouth during the ride there. Would they want me? I'd already been rejected by a coach of their caliber. It was entirely possible that these coaches would take a pass on me as well. More daunting than being rejected was the notion that I could be accepted.

They were notoriously rough on their girls. They screamed and cursed, threw things. It was even rumored that Parkette coaches had slapped a girl or two. Of course, the whisperings were of swift whacks to the back of the thighs, not punches or face slaps. I dismissed these rumors as likely false or, if true, minor offenses. My parents weren't privy to this sort of gossip; we kept these things amongst ourselves, knowing parents might intervene if they heard everything there was to hear.

Beyond mere talk of abuse, the Strausses' rigor when it came to weight was notorious. The girls weren't allowed to eat anything. We snuck them food at competitions—illicit bagels for sustenance, punishable candy for celebrations. It was known that they weighed their girls twice a day, before and after practice. I would become all too familiar with the drill. Each day, I would be required to step on the scale. I'd tiptoe cautiously toward it, treating it with the fear and reverence it demanded. I'd mount with trepidation, exhaling, praying lightness. Fingers euphemistically crossed, I'd wish a half pound less, even a quarter, just to meet with a wink of approval. Otherwise, there'd be punishment. Weight gain meant more workout, running and jumping swathed in a rubbery sweat suit designed to burn off unsightly pounds. And, of course, there was shame. At Parkettes, there was nothing more shameful than gaining weight.

The Parkettes competed in white leotards to display how little fat they carried. Their stomach muscles carved ripples beneath the Lycra. Their hip bones popped, bold and pointy. These coaches were intent on having the thinnest girls on the competition floor. On my first day, I feared I could be rejected on these grounds alone.

Hiding the blister I'd chewed into my lip on the car ride from New Jersey, I entered the gym with my mom. She gave a nod of encouragement, but she was clearly nervous as well.

She, too, wanted to make the cut. She wanted to be the mom of a girl good enough to make Parkettes. Good enough to dream of the Olympics.

The gym was grand. It was vast and fully equipped with the latest training implements. The boys' team—more masculinely called Gymnastrum—trained to the right, relegated to a quarter of the total space. The girls got the rest. A foam pit ran the length of the back. Each event had a station that led to the pit, for learning new skills safely. A vault runway dumped girls into it, two sets of bars were poised above it, a balance beam for dismount practice was perched near its edge, and of course there were several tumbling strips that led to the cushy foam. Lolo's gym didn't even have one of these extravagant training devices. This was luxurious, state-of-the-art. There were scores of beams, all padded, the latest variety. At Will-Moor we fought for the padded beams, and if we lost, we were relegated to the hard and slippery wooden ones. There were enough sets of uneven parallel bars that each girl in a training group could have her own. This meant no breaks waiting for another girl to go. There were two whole forty-by-forty-inch floor exercise mats. The warehouse ceilings were so high, the square footage so impressive, that the chalk dust didn't hang in the air, as it did in most gyms. It was a palatial factory. It churned out champions.

Donna Strauss approached, welcoming us with open arms. She hugged me, oddly affectionate, given the reports. She seemed happy to see me. Surprisingly, there would not be a test. The Strausses had seen me compete for the last two years. They'd witnessed my impressive sweep at the New Jersey invitational meet. They wanted me. Perhaps because they had recently fallen in status—they had no girls qualify for the 1984 Olympic Team—they were less picky than they'd been in the past when they could have had their choice among the best.

They were rebuilding, looking for "good deals": able, hardworking girls of moderate ability whom they could turn into something special.

Mrs. Strauss presented the gym, suggested I put my things in a locker and start workout with the girls. My mom took a seat in the balcony to which all parents were relegated. At least the ones who were allowed to remain in the gym to watch. My mother was granted special privileged "watcher" status, on that day and all future days, because of the distance we drove. She couldn't be expected to wander the streets of Allentown aimlessly while I trained for seven hours. But many parents were banned from the gym entirely. The coaches rationalized that some girls just couldn't concentrate with their eagle-eyed parents on the premises. More likely, the coaches knew that they should hide their behavior from as many parents as possible.

Another Jennifer showed me to the locker room. I followed shyly, feeling inferior. She was so skinny, almost hollowed haunches where I had pudge. There was a flat plateau from her upper leg to her lower back. Above that, her ribs were visible, rippling beneath her bodysuit, starkly pronounced. From the back. I could see her ribs from the back. I resolved not to remove my running tights, usually just worn during warm-ups, for the entirety of practice. I emptied my bladder, removed my shoes, and placed them in an empty locker. I pulled my tights over my leotard and followed Jen back into the gym.

The other girls were already working out. Cindy and Nicole, the impressive pixies I'd seen a few years earlier at Parkettes camp, were already gone, having left the sport at thirteen, before starting high school. The youngest Parkettes—the new stars—were on beam. These ten-year-olds—Lisa, Marsha, and Jane—would be attempting to qualify for elite this year. They were all performing advanced tumbling runs, skills that

I'd never attempted. They lackadaisically threw themselves through triple back handsprings and back handspring layout series, sometimes hitting and often falling. I watched, amazed, as they kept going, throwing ten, twenty, thirty without stopping.

Off the bat, I was adopted by an assistant coach, John. I would become his pet, making good on my pattern of always being favored by the second in command. But they were all so warm and welcoming. They set about endearing themselves to me, a prerequisite, in order to wield complete control in the long run. They were manipulative parents. They lavished me with enthusiasm and encouragement. Knowing if they took it away, showed disappointment in me later, I would pine for just a nod, a wink of validation. And I'd be willing to do almost anything to get it.

The Strausses were an unlikely married couple. Donna was petite, under five feet tall, less than a hundred pounds. She looked remarkably like my mother with her pixie haircut, dark skin, and dark hair. Though she was about forty, she appeared as though she could've been a gymnast herself just a few years earlier, but she never had been. Bill, her husband, was about ten years older than she was. He was balding—his fine hair, worn in a monk's bowl cut, revealed a round shiny spot on the back of his head—and paunchy, which gave him a teddy bear quality. Though he could roar, he was always the first with a hug. He was the dad. Bill didn't coach regularly. He became very attached to certain girls, and when they left or retired or became too injured to take it anymore, he took time off to lick his wounds. He had been on a sabbatical after Gina Stallone (a former World Championship Team member) left for college. He was slowly insinuating himself back into the day-to-day goings-on at Parkettes with the arrival of Hope Spivey. He dipped his toe in the water, coming in during practice for an hour or two at first, just to coach Hope through a new tumbling skill. She was a spitfire from West Virginia. A diamond in the rough, Hope had raw athletic talent with little grace, poise, or control. She brought Bill back into the fold. He only coached his favorites, after all, and Hope's youthful exuberance (she was barely thirteen) and sheer potential drew his interest. During my tenure, Bill would spend negligible time coaching me. The modicum of attention he would turn my way brought a shine to my demeanor. He's the only person who has ever called me Jenny. I've never fit the diminutive and "cute" bill of a Jenny. But I liked it when he did it. I basked in its endearment.

Then there was Robin. Thirtyish, blond, and muscular, she had been a national team member in the seventies, coached by the Strausses. She owed her early success to them as well as her current employed status. In blue-collar Allentown—home of the downsized Mack trucks and Bethlehem Steel—a stable job was coveted. Robin needed the Parkettes. She didn't have a college degree, and her husband was often out of work. She had three kids—a son and twin baby girls. The babies sat nearby in a playpen while she coached. Robin was the only full-time coach I ever had who had actually done women's gymnastics. She could be sadistically harsh with us girls because her livelihood depended on it. Our success was her survival.

Finally, there was John. He was tall, rangy, goofy-looking. He had buckteeth, bulging eyes, thick glasses. He wore a denim leisure suit when he got dressed up for special occasions. John had never been a gymnast. He'd played volleyball in college. I will never understand how someone who has never done the sport makes a career as a gymnastics coach. The need for an income is comprehensible, but why not choose something with which one has personal experience? How can a coach explain the how-tos of the uneven bars when he has never attempted a giant swing or a release move? How can he provide direction on overcoming fear when he's never done it himself? Even if a male coach is a former gymnast, he has practiced an entirely different sport from his girl students. He knows little about how to tumble on a four-inch-wide balance beam. Different events, different tricks. It's like a former swimmer coaching track and field. Both races require swiftness, but does a swimmer know how to explain the ways of speed on land?

I always knew something else was at play. These men coach young, prepubescent girls in leotards, touch their nearly naked bodies as they fly through the air. They guide them to safety as they grab them, manhandling their immature bodies. John was lewd and lascivious. Despite being married, he flirted with all the women who came into his field of vision. But he didn't exhibit any inappropriate inclinations with the girls on the Parkettes team. He may have liked being near all the barely dressed teens, but he never explicitly let on. He never crossed a line. Unlike Patrick, the coach I knew from Parkettes camp, years earlier. Patrick was no longer with the club by the time I arrived. He'd been asked to leave quietly, embroiled in accusations of inappropriate behavior toward some of the younger girls, those who'd always been his obvious favorites. With John, there was a constant semi-sexual tension. But he was protective of us. He knew others, like Patrick, crossed the line, and he prided himself on never having done so. He may have liked looking, but he would never touch. And he harbored grave ire for those who did, likely angered by their weakness.

I know that John genuinely believed in me and wanted me to succeed in gymnastics, more than any other coach had. Lolo may have wanted to fashion me into a strong woman, guide me toward adulthood. But John wanted me to be a winner. He was the first coach who truly saw me as a potential champion.

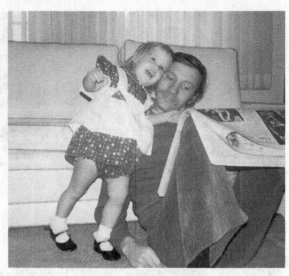

Jennifer with her father, 1970.

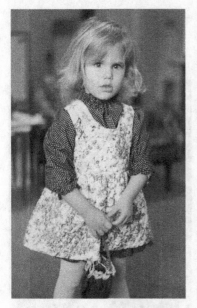

Jennifer, as a "Joey Heatherton look-alike," Turkey, 1973.

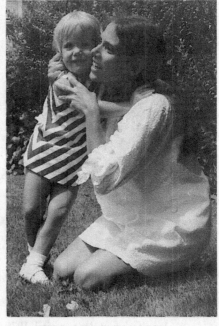

Jennifer with her mother who is expecting Chris, 1971.

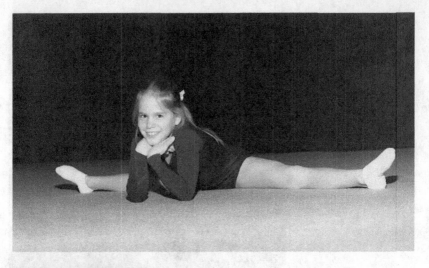

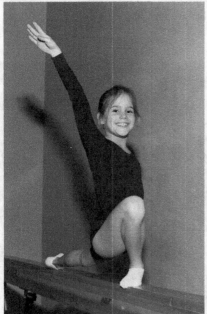

Jennifer, as a member of the Cabrielles, 1977.

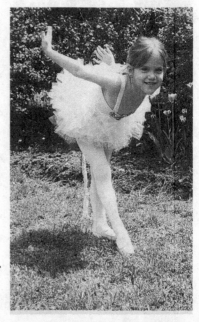

Jennifer's first dance recital, 1975.

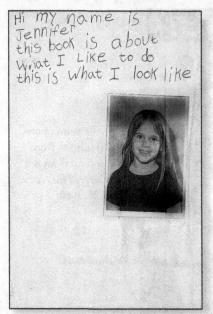

Hi my name is Jennifer this book is about what I Like to do this is what I look like

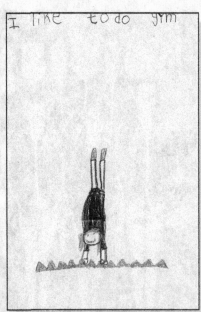

I like to do gym

A kindergarten art project, "I love gym," 1976.

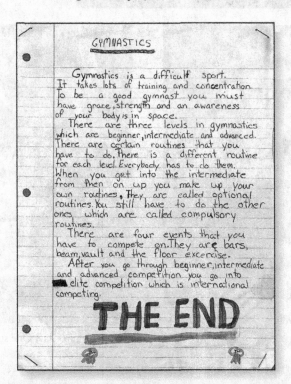

GYMNASTICS

Gymnastics is a difficult sport. It takes lots of training and concentration. To be a good gymnast you must have grace, strength and an awareness of your body is in space.

There are three levels in gymnastics which are beginner, intermediate and advanced. There are certain routines that you have to do. There is a different routine for each level. Everybody has to do them. When you get into the intermediate from then on up you make up your own routines. They are called optional routines. You still have to do the other ones which are called compulsory routines.

There are four events that you have to compete on. They are bars, beam, vault and the floor exercise.

After you go through beginner, intermediate and advanced competition you go into elite competition which is international competing.

THE END

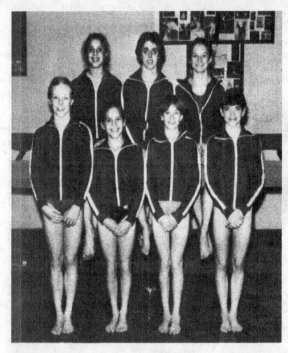

Cabrielle team photo, 1980 (Jennifer, front row, second from left), *The Cherry Hill News*, April 24, 1980.

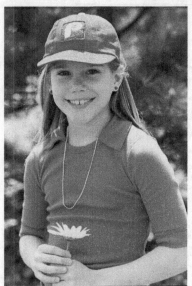

Jennifer, 1980.

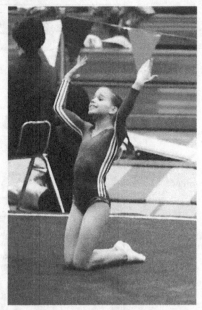

Competing in Class One states, 1979.

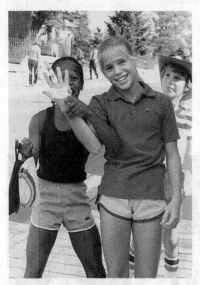

With Angie, at nationals in New Mexico, 1981.

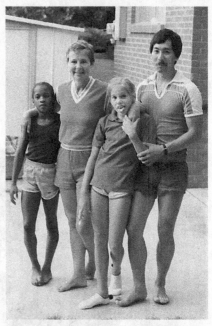

At nationals, 1981 (from left: Angie, Lolo, Jennifer, Wes).

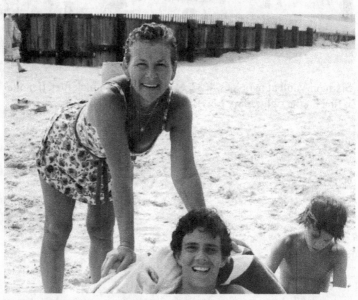

Visiting Lolo at her beach house, 1981 (from left: Lolo, Merle Sey, and Chris Sey).

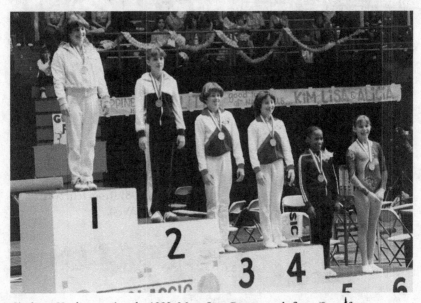

Sixth on Vault at nationals, 1982. Mary Lou Retton took first. (Jennifer is first on the right; Mary Lou Retton is atop the podium.)

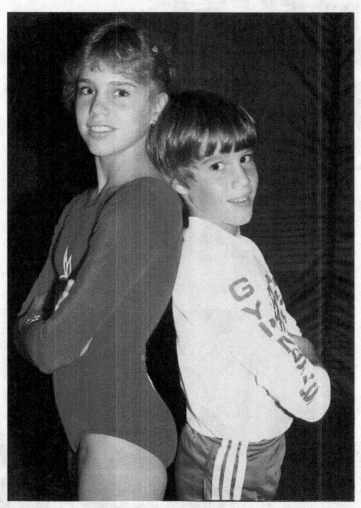

At Will-Moor with Chris, 1981.

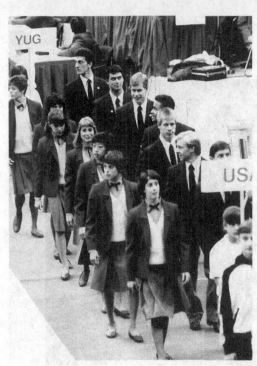

Opening Ceremonies, 1985 World Championships.

The fall at 1985 World Championships.

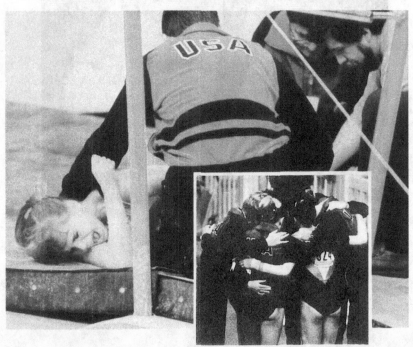

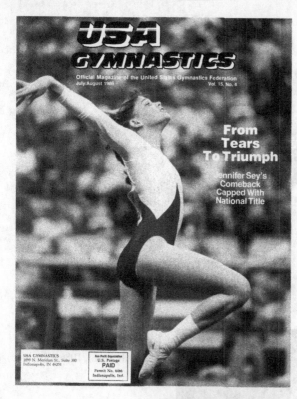

On the cover of
*USA Gymnastics*, July/
August 1986 issue.

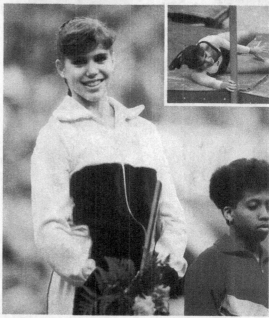

"Mending Broken
Dreams: Disaster in
Montreal Transforms
to Triumph in
Indianapolis," *USA
Gymnastics* cover story,
July/August 1986 issue.

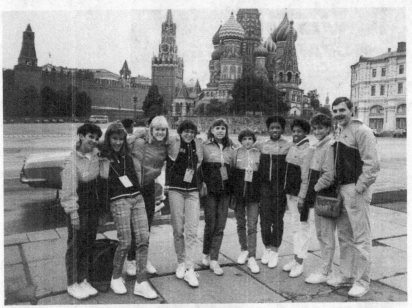

In Moscow for the Good Will Games with the U.S. team, 1986.

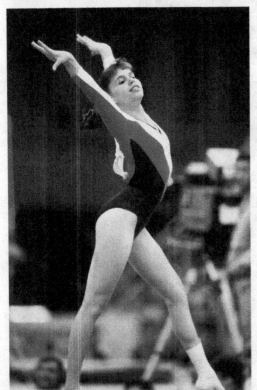

Competing on floor exercise at the Good Will Games, 1986.

April 7, 1987

**United States Gymnastics Federation**

1099 N. Meridian St.
Suite 380
Indianapolis, IN 46204
(317) 638-8743
Telex: 27-2585 USGYM-IND

Ms. Jennifer Sey
1517 W. Congress
Allentown, PA 18102

Dear Jennifer:

On behalf of the United States Gymnastics Federation, please accept our congratulations on being selected the United States Olympic Committee's Gymnast of the Year. This is a tremendous honor and something you should be very proud of.

I know you have a very busy schedule and I want to thank you for taking time to come to Indianapolis to participate in the ceremonies surrounding this award. I hope you enjoyed the evening and your brief stay in Indianapolis. I was very pleased that you were able to come and represent our sport.

Jennifer, your accomplishments this past year are a real tribute to your dedication and commitment. I know you would have great success during your participation in all of the exciting events that are coming up in 1987 and 1988. All of us at the USGF wish you the very best in your endeavors.

Once again, Jennifer, congratulations! We all look forward to the excitement in the future of your gymnastics career.

For the United States Gymnastics Federation,
Sincerely,

Mike Jacki
Executive Director

mj/lab

cc: Executive Committee
    Kathy Kelly

The United States Olympic Committee letter that announced Jennifer had been named the "United States Olympic Committee's Gymnast of the Year," April 7, 1987.

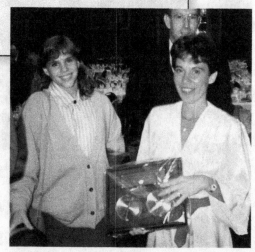

Awarded Athlete of the Year, 1987 (with Donna Strauss).

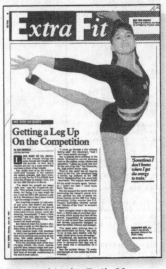

Featured in the *Daily News*,
April 20, 1987.

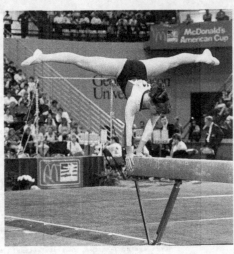

Competing at the American Cup, 1987.

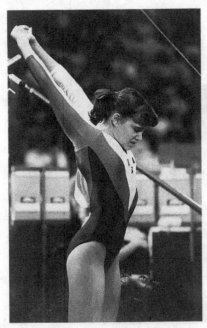

Preparing for competition on the bars,
American Cup 1987.

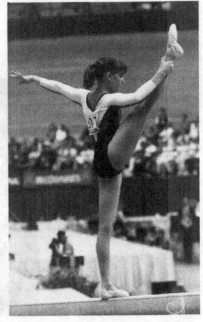

Competing on the beam, American
Cup, 1987.

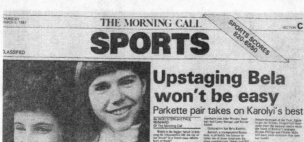

# SPORTS

SPORTS SCORES 820-6550

## Upstaging Bela won't be easy
### Parkette pair takes on Karolyi's best

By JACK STEIN and PAUL REINHARD
Of The Morning Call

"Upstaging Bela won't be easy: Parkette pair takes on Karolyi's best," (Jennifer, right, and Hope Spivey, left) *The Morning Call* (Allentown), March 3, 1987.

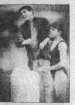

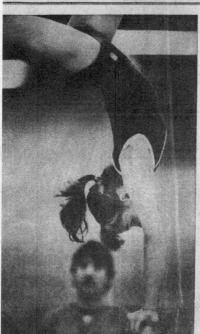

## The Philadelphia Inquirer
### family/home/fashion

section K

Sunday, March 22, 198[7]

## The ups and downs of a young gymnast

*Jennifer Sey, 17, has endured pain and heartache on the way to the top.*

By Karen Heller
Inquirer Staff Writer

*Jennifer and her brother, Christopher*

"The Ups and Downs of a Young Gymnast: Jennifer Sey, 17, has endured pain and heartache on the way to the top," *Philadelphia Inquirer*, March 22, 1987.

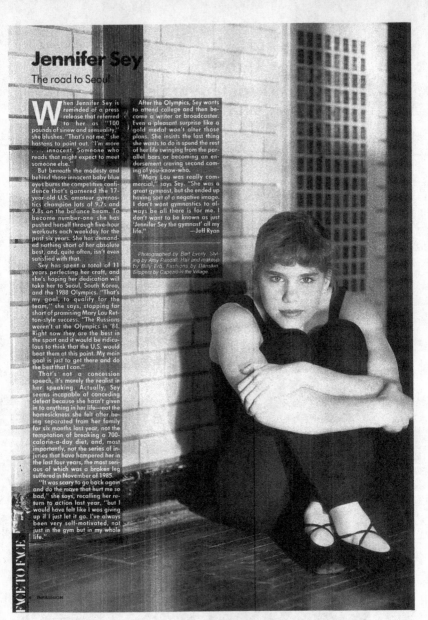

# Jennifer Sey

The road to Seoul

When Jennifer Sey is reminded of a press release that referred to her as "100 pounds of sinew and sensuality," she blushes. "That's not me," she hastens to point out. "I'm more . . . innocent. Someone who reads that might expect to meet someone else."

But beneath the modesty and behind those innocent baby blue eyes burns the competitive confidence that's garnered the 17-year-old U.S. amateur gymnastics champion lots of 9.7s and 9.8s on the balance beam. To become number-one she has pushed herself through five-hour workouts each weekday for the past six years. She has demanded nothing short of her absolute best, and, quite often, isn't even satisfied with that.

Sey has spent a total of 11 years perfecting her craft, and she's hoping her dedication will take her to Seoul, South Korea, and the 1988 Olympics. "That's my goal, to qualify for the team," she says, stopping far short of promising Mary Lou Retton-style success. "The Russians weren't at the Olympics in '84. Right now they are the best in the sport and it would be ridiculous to think that the U.S. would beat them at this point. My main goal is just to get there and do the best that I can."

That's not a concession speech, it's merely the realist in her speaking. Actually, Sey seems incapable of conceding defeat because she hasn't given in to anything in her life—not the homesickness she felt after being separated from her family for six months last year, not the temptation of breaking a 700-calorie-a-day diet, and, most importantly, not the series of injuries that have hampered her in the last four years, the most serious of which was a broken leg suffered in November of 1985.

"It was scary to go back again and do the move that hurt me so bad," she says, recalling her return to action last year, "but I would have felt like I was giving up if I just let it go. I've always been very self-motivated, not just in the gym but in my whole life."

After the Olympics, Sey wants to attend college and then become a writer or broadcaster. Even a pleasant surprise like a gold medal won't alter those plans. She insists the last thing she wants to do is spend the rest of her life swinging from the parallel bars or becoming an endorsement craving second coming of you-know-who.

"Mary Lou was really commercial," says Sey. "She was a great gymnast, but she ended up having sort of a negative image. I don't want gymnastics to always be all there is for me. I don't want to be known as just 'Jennifer Sey the gymnast' all my life."
—Jeff Ryan

*Photographed by Bart Everly. Styling by Amy Randall. Hair and makeup by Billy Erb. Fashions by Danskin. Slippers by Capezio in the Village.*

FACE TO FACE

INFASHION

"Jennifer Sey: The Road to Seoul," *In Fashion* magazine, May/June 1987.

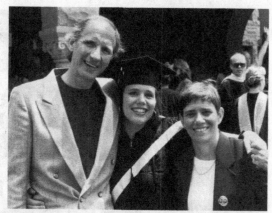

Jennifer, celebrating her graduation from Stanford University with her parents, 1992.

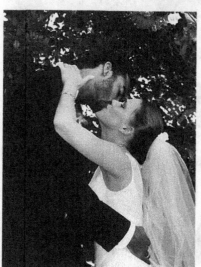

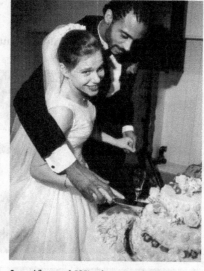

Jennifer and Winslow on their wedding day, September 12, 1999.

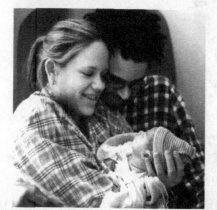

Jennifer and Winslow celebrating the birth of their first son, September 30, 2000.

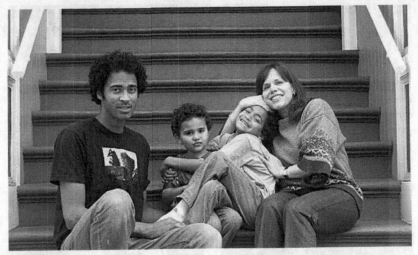

The Warren/Sey family: Winslow, Wyatt, Virgil, and Jennifer , 2007.

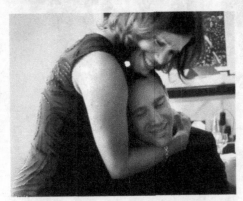

Jennifer with Chris on his wedding day, 2003.

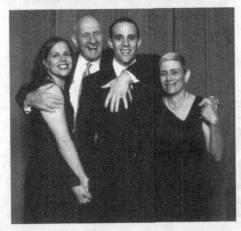

The Sey family: Jennifer, Mark, Chris, and Merle.

Lolo believed I was smart and a truly good person; she believed my tenacity and focus would get me places in life. But she never really believed I was better than Angie, let alone any of the other girls I would need to top in order to win. John knew I was mentally tougher than most, capable of willing myself to win. He had watched me as I transformed myself from a soft-bodied, unexceptional junior national team member to the fierce competitor who stole every event at the recent Garden State Classic. John may have been an "assistant coach," but at Parkettes, each coach had his or her girls. I was his girl.

All of the coaches wanted me to like it at Parkettes, so they took it easy on me at first. Relatively. They needed me to stay, to choose them. They had only recently lost Cindy and Nicole; they needed new young seniors to build their army. Parkettes' strength was in numbers. If they had enough girls in the mix, even if one got hurt, there was another to take her place. If one girl turned out to be a disappointment, or another ended up wanting to go out with boys and go to parties when she got to high school, there was another waiting in the wings. As coaches, they figured it was a sport of odds, to an extent. You play enough hands, you're bound to win eventually.

I was ecstatic. I'd never had so many girls to train with. Or to be friends with. I was an introvert, and miles from cool or popular at my high school. I kept to myself, got A's, didn't drink. I was underdeveloped, socially immature, not interested in boys or sex. But here there were loads of girls just like me. All of them flat-chested and narrow-hipped with no interest in making out or chugging wine coolers. All we wanted to do was get through school each day as quickly as possible, to train for as long as possible. We maintained good grades so that no teacher or parent would ever threaten our shortened school day. Our calendars were determined by competition seasons, not the school year, our milestones measured in competitive rankings ("I didn't win, but I moved up to seventh!"), not sexual exploits ("I went to third base!").

I had found a club that I wanted to be part of, that also wanted me. At least ten of the girls at Parkettes were competing at the elite level, and another ten were training to qualify. Many of the girls boarded in Allentown. Some who lived there, far away from their parents, were as young as ten. The Armstrong family—whose daughter Jessica was a senior elite of modest ranking—housed several gymnasts, up to five at any given time. They crammed the girls into the attic, stuffed with bunk beds in the musty dark, while Jessica enjoyed her perfect little girl's bedroom, flooded with light and pink frilly bedding. Mrs. Armstrong strictly monitored the girls' food intake according to Mrs. Strauss's instructions. Some of the other gymnasts lived with assistant coaches, other families. If I needed to make the move to Allentown, there were plenty of options for living arrangements.

Before I became a Parkette, I was accustomed to attending competitions either alone or with one other girl, Angie. She and I braved it alone. Us against the world, we battled the throngs of Parkette-like teams, fighting for our measly time on the beam during warm-ups. Now I'd have a posse. I'd have confidence in numbers. We'd march into competitions, taking over the floor. Dazzling and immodest in our bright white leotards, our sheer numbers intimidating. We'd clear the floor of girls without squads. We'd be a gang in pincurl ponytails. Heaven.

I had admired cliques of girls in high school, the cheerleading squad identically dressed on game days, sporting their short skirts and lettered sweaters in the halls as they strutted with impudence from class to class. Now I would be part of a squad, I would be part of something bigger than myself. I would be admired, perhaps envied, as I entered the arena, bolstered by identical teammates marching in perfect unison.

After the warm welcome, the Parkettes coaches put me through the rounds. John wanted to see what I could do. We started slowly.

"Why don't you warm up on bars," John said. "Let's see your free-hips. Your Stalders. Your giants." After completing what he termed my "warm-up"—series upon series of connecting swing moves, some stretched out, some in a straddled position—I'd already done more than an entire bar practice at Will-Moor.

"Okay." Not terribly impressed but not ready to throw me out, he pushed me to see what I would try. Guts meant a lot at Parkettes. More than technique. More than athleticism. That's why it was the perfect place for me.

"Let's see your release moves—a Deltchev? Jaeger? What do you got?"

I chalked my hands. I'd been working on all of these moves, had mastered none. I decided to start with Jaegers, the move I was least afraid of.

"Need a spot?"

I shook my head, afraid that accepting would reflect poorly on me, diminishing my bravery in his eyes.

I jumped up to grab the high bar, pulled myself over to a hip-resting position, facing the low bar. I reversed my grip, as is required for this trick. Without pause, I cast my body up to a handstand, swung through, piking my legs to miss the low bar with plenty of space, released, flipped, and caught the bar with a loud crash of my heels against the fiberglass. *Ouch.*

"You okay?" he asked, not really wanting to know.

I nodded, rechalked my hands.

"Again," he said.

Again. Again. Over and over, I swung through the Jaegers, banging my heels on the bar almost every time. He was testing my will as he urged me to allow my body to stay outstretched for a longer time, barely missing the low bar, so as to build more speed, thus generating more height in the flip. I didn't even consider saying no. I didn't want to be rejected from the team. At Will-Moor, I was asked to do things, given the choice of saying no. If I was too scared, I could wait until I felt less so. Wes allowed me to practice drills until my confidence built, or never built. With John and the Parkettes, going when scared was the assumption. The will to achieve no matter what the level of fear was the price of entry into elite gymnastics.

So I kept going. I let my body stay stretched in a perfectly straight line for longer and longer, barely bending in time to miss the low bar, each time crashing my heels into the bar on the way down. I'd crash them again upon completion of the flip, on the high bar, when catching. By the end of my bar practice I had two egg-sized lumps on the backs of my heels, just below the Achilles tendon. John offered to tape foam blocks to the afflicted area, but I declined. I could handle it. After the Jaegers, we went on to Deltchevs, another release move. I had practiced this one far less, so I accepted his offer for a spot. Without pause, I performed one after another, ultimately going it alone without his assistance. I'd never done that before. With all of Lolo's coaching, cajoling, I'd never feared her, never craved her approval enough to set my fear aside. There was no need.

On floor, he wanted to see my layout pike, a double back with the first somersault outstretched, the second with the legs pulled toward the body. I performed this regularly in competition.

"Do the whole thing laid out," he challenged. I winced. "Try," he coaxed.

I didn't want to disappoint him. No coach had ever asked me to try something this difficult. Even at Karolyi's camp, when the instructors asked other girls to try this one, they never asked me. Gary God-son wouldn't even let me get near a trick like this. He'd barely let me watch Angie do it, relegating me to the corner, drilling rudimentary lead-ins. This was my big chance.

John hurled me through it. He tossed me with all his might. I know this because I landed on my feet. And this was a move that was well beyond my capabilities. He wanted me to feel what it felt like to do something that spectacular. He wanted me to feel what it felt like to be the best. I soared.

Swept up in the promise of new moves learned, my dad made good on his word to purchase a van. He bought a great big one, complete with a desk for studying, a groovy stripe on the outside, and plush tan carpet that could make a comfortable bed if I needed to steal a nap. My mom wedged herself behind the wheel each weekday and drove me, almost two hours each way, to Parkettes to train. A paid driver or my dad took an odd day here and there, allowing my mom some time with Chris, who still trained at Will-Moor. (Most days Chris was driven to and from practice by an older boy on his team and was left to look after himself in the afternoons before pickup.) Each day at noon I was picked up from Haddonfield High School, where I was a sophomore. The state of New Jersey excused me from school early, permitting me to skip lunch, study hall, and gym. Exceptions were made for students with special aptitudes.

Together, my mom and I made the trip up the northwest-bound highway to Allentown. I'd eat my lunch and finish nearly all of my trigonometry and chemistry homework in the car on the way there. By the time we pulled up in front of the rainbow-painted gym (it screamed, "We have fun in here!"), my legs were cramped and I was sleepy.

We'd arrive around two-thirty. The other girls had already been working out for at least an hour and a half. They were all dismissed from the local public and Catholic schools at twelve-thirty, the same arrangement made with the local Allentown schools that I had in New Jersey. But the drive time put me behind. I was trying to ingratiate myself with the coaches and integrate with the girls, but being off schedule made it difficult. I was often in a "rotation" (the training group of girls who went from event to event together) by myself because of my late start. It made it difficult to feel completely part of the team.

The coaches excused my tardiness in the beginning, another way of taking it easy on me, to forge the relationship. Ultimately, they must have known that I'd beg my parents to let me move to Allentown. They counted on the fact that I'd get tired of not being part of the team's rhythm, of always feeling behind in missing an hour of practice up front. They knew that racing to cram it all in, toiling after the other girls were wrapping up, and forcing my mom to drive the winding highway late at night would wear me down. Arriving home at 10:00 P.M., going straight to bed, and then doing it all over again would get tiresome. Their patience was all part of the indoctrination.

We did this five days a week, my mom and I. The local girls and the boarders who lived far from home went to the gym on Saturdays, too, only Sundays allotted for rest. I didn't practice on the weekends at all. I was grateful to forgo the four hours in the car but panicky about missing valuable practice time and falling even further behind.

My family revolved around my new path. All of the adults in my circle colluded to support the cause—becoming a winning gymnast. Teachers excused my absences; my parents' friends willingly pitched in to help with my brother; even Lolo stepped aside graciously to support my dream. If I needed to go to Parkettes—train six hours a day, drive a hundred miles each way, stay engaged with schoolwork just enough to maintain my grades—then all generally rational adults would comply. Winning was everything, after all. And my brother, well, he'd just need to fend for himself. I never questioned it.

# PART III

1987

I HAVE COME BACK TO HIDE. I AM SQUIRRELED AWAY IN THIS hole of a gym, hiding from the Gymnastics Federation, the national team, the coaches who matter, the competitions that I will embarrass myself in. The federation officials are calling to see whether I will attend the upcoming World Championships. I qualified months ago, before my body retreated, refusing me in the only thing I've ever known. I have crawled into this cave to die.

I pretend to work out. I drive to the gym each day, arriving later and later with every week that passes. I consider not going to practice, sitting in the mall parking lot and eating trail mix with sickly sweet yogurt almonds and dried pineapple (junk food masquerading as health food) until my throat is coated with sugar and I feel like I'm going to vomit. I don't throw up; I swallow laxatives instead. Somehow this seems less egregious, less sick. I can just pretend that tomorrow's diarrhea is a function of too much bad food rather than the gulping of boxes of pills.

I finally show up at the gym. I get there despite the fact that I consider pulling across the median, driving into oncoming traffic on Route 295. Once I arrive, I stretch for an unnecessarily long time. An hour of sitting in a straddle position, motionless, until my feet grow numb. I sit close to the mirror looking at my face, slack and tired and gaining pudge around the cheeks and chin. I am not the girl I was two years ago. Or even two months ago, before I left Parkettes. The former national champion is lost amidst the disappointment. Just two years piled on, but I am heavy with the weight of aging, failure, and being left behind. I am eighteen. But I feel like I am a hundred years old, my body aches. I am so tired.

I finally drag myself from the floor exercise mat, my legs stiff from having sat in a split for too long. I move onto beam, the only event my nonexistent energy level can handle. I warm up with a few split leaps, some turns. These simple moves are difficult for me now. I wobble, fall sometimes. Then it's time to move on to the real tricks. I used to perform tumbling runs. Two back handsprings to a layout back somersault. Sometimes two no-handed layouts in a row. I'd land without a wobble. I could do ten, twenty, without a mistake. Now I'm afraid to do a single back handspring, a trick I've been able to do since I was seven years old. I bend my knees to go, but my head tells me to stop. I can't picture it, it seems impossible that my hands would actually land on the beam if I were to rotate my body 180 degrees, backward into a handstand. I bend my legs to jump, like I've done millions of times before, but this time, my mind screeches to a halt. I step backward to stop my momentum. But my body is almost airborne, light without the pull of gravity. I've propelled myself and I can't completely stop. My back foot misses the beam, and I land on my tailbone, roll to my back on the beam, and then crash to the floor. That will be it for me today.

Lolo crawls over to me underneath the beam. I lie there, too tired to even cry. I am curled into a ball, and she gathers me in her arms. "You are the 1986 national champion. You always will be. Don't you ever forget that."

But it doesn't matter. Who cares? I bury my face in her chest, and she rocks and rocks and rocks until I finally cry. She mothers me the way my own mother can't because she is too lost in disappointment and self-pity. My mother gave everything so that I could do this. My dreams became hers, and then I didn't have them anymore, but she did. My mother is still holding her daughter's dreams, and she has nowhere to put them. She wants to give them back, but I don't want them anymore.

Lolo sends me home for the day. She does not expect anything from me other than to try to get happy again. To move on. To make it through until September when I can accept my position as a freshman at Stanford. She doesn't care that my body and my mind are failing me. She knows that I will find them again.

I will slink away from the sport of gymnastics unable to feel pride in my past accomplishments because the entire affair has ended with such humiliation. My career—once celebrated as the exemplification of triumph over adversity—is now a blight that I will carry with me. It is a sore that becomes easily irritated. In my quiet, dark moments, I will be reminded of my failure to stick it out. To barrel through. To stay on top and make the Olympics.

It will chafe every time I fail at something, no matter how small. When I am passed over for a promotion at work, the wound will fester. When I can't get through the birth of my first son without the relief of an epidural, it will inflame. When

I give up nursing my children before the full year recommended by pediatricians, I will be reminded of this obsession to be the best and then fail to be. And when I am reminded of the thing itself—"You were a gymnast?" "Yes." "Were you in the Olympics?" "No."—it will torment most of all. My inability to stay the course, to make it through to the 1988 Olympics, will be proof of my undeservingness. It is a ridiculous shame—and the shame begets more shame because I can't get over it. I can't get over having been the best and then failing to be anymore. It waits to be revealed, to remind me it is there, with the slightest provocation. It will sit there, deep in my gut, no matter what else I accomplish, for the rest of my life.

# 1985–1989

# Chapter 17

I LOST WEIGHT RIGHT AWAY AT Parkettes. The training sessions were so much more rigorous, it was inevitable. Five pounds were shed without a thought. Though I wasn't trying, I was pleased with the results. I was molding a gymnast's body from what I now understood to be my previously amorphous form. I felt sure Karolyi would want me, if he saw the way I looked. But he would be too late; his lack of foresight had prompted me to find another home.

Because the coaches were satisfied with my weight loss, they didn't comment on my eating habits. Until, one day, after practice, around seven-thirty, my mom offered me a bagel with cream cheese and the standard diet soda. I stood by the office, where my mom had already started helping out, waiting to go home. I was eating my bagel while she finished chatting with the other office moms. The girls eyed me, appalled, as they headed toward the exit. They would never eat in front of our coaches. I hadn't learned this lesson yet and didn't think anything of it. It was just a bagel. And I was hungry. These were the days when carbohydrates were encouraged for athletes. I was confused by the suggestion that maybe I should curtail the eating of energy-producing foods after a seven-hour workout. I'd already started limiting my food intake before practice to avoid extra pounds on the scale caused by the simple weight of food in my stomach. So in the evening, I was famished. I licked the cream cheese and gnawed the bagel while I sipped my soda.

"You gonna eat *all* of that?" John's eyes, distorted by his thick glasses, didn't scold. They danced to ease the censure.

"Sure." I took another bite.

"Why don't you save half?"

I paused. He was serious. I wrapped my bagel back up in the aluminum foil. "I'm not hungry anymore." My stomach growled.

He knocked on the office window to get my mom's attention. He snatched the bagel from my hand, waving it toward her. "What are you doin', givin' her a whole bagel? With cream cheese!"

My mom couldn't hear him through the glass. She smiled. He tossed the remaining half of the bagel into the trash. My mom came out of the office. "What?" She laughed, as eager for his approval as I was.

John put an arm around her. She melted into him. "What are you doing, a whole bagel?" he said again. He smiled all the while, feigning lightheartedness.

"I don't know." She giggled, conceding that she'd made a mistake in not objecting.

We got home late that night. I went right to bed, no dinner. My half bagel lay heavy in my empty stomach while John's deft but hefty admonishment weighed on my remorseful conscience.

My weight wasn't all that dropped when I started Parkettes. My grades suffered, too. The daily car trips took their toll. I got my first B on a chemistry test. It didn't concern me. I was still going to get an A in the class. I knew that other kids, even those in honors chemistry, got B's all the time. But my teacher noticed a change. She asked me to stay after class one day.

"Is something happening at home?" she asked.

I shook my head, not offering a verbal response, not really sure why she'd delayed me. My grades were still above average.

"I've noticed your grades. They're slipping. And you missed a homework assignment." I shrugged. "You look a little tired," she said.

"I have a meet coming up." They all knew I was a gymnast. They didn't realize it was a different level of commitment than the high school team.

"You're sure that's all?" she pressed. I nodded.

Again I felt chastised. I took her concerned words as condemnation. I wasn't worried she would tell my parents. It was too big of a school to be concerned about that kind of personal interaction. Besides, even if she had the initiative to call them, my parents wouldn't fall prey to worry. They wouldn't be concerned about a single B limiting my college choices. I was only a sophomore, had achieved straight A's to date, and had an outstanding extracurricular schedule that would undoubtedly enable me to get into a respectable school, when the time came. They wouldn't require that we rethink commuting to Parkettes. But my face burned with humiliation as I vowed to myself that I would maintain A's to avoid this kind of unwanted attention from a teacher. Just like in the gym, I only wanted to be called out for doing something better than the other kids. To be noticed for screwing up was mortifying for such a devout perfectionist. I hugged my books close to my chest and kept my eyes on the ground as I found my way to my next class.

With the strain of daily four-hour car trips and an hour of missed practice each day, I decided it was time to move to Allentown. We'd been commuting for only a few months when my parents relented, yet another sacrifice in support of my pursuit. They'd seen such improvement in my capability already. I'd mastered several new release moves on bars, a tumbling series on balance beam, and was working toward a Tsukahara with a full twist on vault, valued at a 10. To start off with a 10 improved my chances of getting a score in the mid-9s, which would guarantee a higher placement in the upcoming nationals. In the past, all of my vaults were valued at a 9.7. Unlikely near perfection was required to post a score in the mid-9s. The "Tsuk" full was going to be my saving grace. I'd learned as much in the half year I'd spent at Parkettes as I'd learned in four years at Lolo's. The intensity of the workouts and the ferocious ardor of the coaches were paying off. What might I do if I got that extra hour of practice in every day, an extra Saturday workout, a little more sleep? I'd be a force.

It was decided that I would move in with Beth and her four-year-old son, Wes. Beth was a coach at Parkettes, but she taught only the youngest team girls, the seven- and eight-year-olds. She was not involved in my training, which made it a suitable living situation, according to my parents. At least at "home" I'd be relieved from the pressures of the coaches.

I moved into her modest suburban three-bedroom house on a gray Sunday evening. She'd been awarded the house in her recent divorce, but her hourly wage and inconsistent alimony payments made it difficult to afford the mortgage. My parents agreed to pay three hundred dollars a month to cover any expenses associated with my boarding, offsetting some of her costs in the process. They dropped me off with all of my things, moved me into Beth's spare bedroom, and drove back to New Jersey. I held back tears as they drove away. It had been my decision, after all. I couldn't make them doubt leaving me there. They'd have stuffed me right back into the car and driven me home. They would have been more than happy to continue the commute, though it must have been a strain on their marriage. With my mom always in the car on her way to and from Allentown, they never saw each other. And while they overlooked their time spent apart due to my gymnastics, they would never have knowingly ignored my despair. To continue training at Parkettes and campaigning for national recognition, I had to hide any distress from my parents.

On that gloomy Sunday night and all subsequent Sundays, I was exiled to Beth's guest room, in a cold house without any of the familiar comforts of home. From now on, these comforts—meals, heat, conversation—were to be enjoyed only on the weekends when I visited my family. Beth's house went unheated most of the time. I took to sleeping in layers and layers of clothes, including mittens and a woolen hat, to ward off the sharp, frosty air. The blankets were scratchy, the towels were thin, and the house was virtually silent. And always dark. The food was appalling and available in only the smallest portions. Beth's own eating disorder, her fear of being held accountable for my weight, and a tenuous financial situation kept the cupboards mostly bare. When stocked, it was with foods unfamiliar or just unpalatable to me: limp bologna, undercooked chicken with a slimy, soupy coating, bright orange processed cheese in the plastic sleeves, canned string beans. The homey meals my mother prepared were a thing of the past. Beth would single-handedly turn me against dinner.

I took to locking myself in my room, a somber, windowless space that barely fit a twin bed. I didn't have a radio or television to keep me company, to break the heavy, wintry silence. I stuck to studying and sleeping. It was quiet and joyless. I was hungry all the time. I retreated into myself, fending off the loneliness with calorie counting and dreams of victory.

I didn't tell my parents about the situation because that would cause them to worry. They might even pull me from Beth's entirely, which would impede my lengthened, more rigorous training schedule. I didn't tell them I needed additional blankets or food because that would prompt questions about the living situation. "Is it cold? Why is it so cold? Are you eating enough? *Are you all right?*" If they asked me these things, I would crack. If they saw me cry, that would be the end of Parkettes for me. They wouldn't tolerate avoidable misery. We were in the trial phase, not yet addicted to high national rankings, newspaper headlines, and covers of *USA Gymnastics* magazine. They would have been willing to call it quits, to go back to the comfort of Lolo's. I just told them everything was fine.

But, in the midst of my false reports, I became a different person. It was during this time at Beth's that I peeled a new gymnast self away from my former child self. A girl divided in two, I teased apart a dedicated, somber, fearless girl from a formerly ambitious but cheerful one. This new girl didn't consider physical comfort or emotional happiness, only winning. She didn't tell her parents about the things that troubled her. She ignored hunger, pain, fear, and loneliness. She developed habits to ward off these unpleasant feelings—dieting and deeply involved body checks. These nightly exams included rib counting and fat pinching to measure diminished and newly lean areas, like the back of the arm, the back of the knee. She measured the distance between her thighs when she stood, the width of her wrists with the thumb and forefinger of the opposite hand. She exercised constantly, dropping to the floor for sit-ups and push-ups in between writing school papers and completing her trigonometry homework. And she slept. In sleep, she felt peaceful, though she often woke in the night, either from the cold or in a panic about weigh-ins the next day. This new girl was humorless and withdrawn. She was out of reach. She kept any sadness hidden, masked with a sober demeanor that could easily be construed as no-nonsense commitment. For anyone who wanted to see it that way.

When I moved to Allentown midway through the school semester during sophomore year, I enrolled in Swain, a small private school with only a handful of other kids in my grade. It was my second high school to date. And as much as I didn't like the first one because I felt out of place, I liked this one even less. It was dark and cold, boring. The kids were all awkward; they could never have survived in a normal public high school. Being surrounded by outsiders only served to reflect my own outsider status. It didn't make me feel like I fit in.

Each morning Mrs. Kuroda picked me up at Beth's and deposited me at school along with her daughters, Missy and Andie, fellow Parkettes. My mom arranged it with Mrs. Kuroda, like carpooling moms do, only my mother never had to drive because she lived two hours away in New Jersey. The Allentown residents regularly volunteered to help the girls who boarded there. It was all a part of being in the Parkette community. The Kuroda girls hated Swain as much as I did. But our parents, who considered themselves above the blue-collar fray of Allentown, saw it as the only viable college-preparatory educational option in this town where the public high school offered vo-tech (employment in automotive repair, carpentry, metalworking) as a means of getting a high school diploma.

After my year of near normalcy at a big public school, Swain was punishment. I wore a uniform—a navy blue blazer adorned with the school's crest and a gray flannel skirt—as I endured one class after the other in the same bleak classroom with the same nerdy kids, no socializing. While I never went in big for any of the school-spirit stuff at Haddonfield High, I felt safer knowing it was there, providing options for an alternate reality. I ended up liking Haddonfield High more than my alternative private elementary school. It made being a conventional teenager an option, if I ever decided that that was what I wanted. It allowed glimpses of what it might be like. If I decided I wanted to go to a football game on Friday night, giggle with the other fourteen- and fifteen-year-old girls about which guy was cutest, if I wanted to go to a pep rally and make fun of the cheerleaders while simultaneously wanting to be one, I could. I could try out for the tennis team, drill team, debate club. I could join the yearbook committee or the school newspaper staff. I could even find myself a boyfriend. That wasn't true at The Philadelphia School, and it definitely wasn't true at Swain. There were six kids in my tenth-grade class, only one boy. Each one was more socially inept and shy than the next. They made *me* feel cool.

I passed the time there, just to get to the gym. Mrs. Kuroda picked us up from school at around 12:30 and dropped us off at the gym by 12:45. That's when the day began. I shook the cold from my bones and prepared for a productive workout. But before we started, there were weigh-ins. I relished stepping on the scale. With the dearth of edible food at Beth's, I continued to shed weight, trimming my already lean body to ninety-five pounds, a feat I never thought possible at a well-muscled five feet three. My eating, or lack of it, was beginning to border on obsessive, each calorie recorded and totaled for the day, never to exceed eight hundred. Over time, the calorie count would dwindle as my underweight body became harder to maintain. But, so far it had been relatively easy. I didn't like the food that was available to me, and it was fun to see the numbers on the scale drop. I was rewarded with appreciative smiles. The coaches could see a gymnast forming, as if carved from a shapeless slab of stone. I basked in their pride. Their approval seduced me. It was all I needed to fuel my self-destruction.

After practice I'd ride home with Beth. She'd serve up one of her slimy pale meals, and I'd push it around on my plate before retiring to my room, stomach growling but hip bones proudly jutting. I'd layer on my clothes for the night—tights, sweat pants, scarf—and set to my homework, determined to maintain my grades, keeping parents and teachers out of my business. And the distraction helped me fend off the dizzying hunger.

When I heard Beth climb the steps, put Wes to bed, and then lock herself in her own room, I'd sometimes tiptoe downstairs to see what snacks I could find to stave off sleep-prohibitive stomach growling. Once, I'd hoped to find peanut butter sandwich cookies, having seen her bring them in from a trip to the grocery store that very evening. I spied her placing them in a cabinet beneath the kitchen sink next to the cleaning supplies, an odd place for food. I assumed they weren't for me, as she was hiding them rather than placing them in plain view in the pantry. When I snuck down to steal one, I couldn't find them, though I'd seen them just hours before. They were gone, an empty box in the trash. I realized she must have devoured them all herself in a fit of bulimic binging. Still intent on finding a treat, I unearthed a stash of forgotten butterscotch chips, dusty and discolored with age. It was a quarter of a bag, maybe three ounces, and I allowed myself only three chips, a late-night snack to tide me over until the morning. I hid the bag behind a sack of flour to ensure it would be there when I returned. With the sugary sweetness lingering on my tongue, I went back up the stairs, mittens pulled on before lights out.

At Beth's I went to bed earlier than I ever had in my life. I'd been a night owl since I was five, when I cajoled my parents into letting me watch *Candid Camera* at ten o'clock. But now I courted sleep because it kept the loneliness at bay. I didn't feel the bone-chilling cold when I was sleeping. I didn't miss my mom and dad. I didn't have a headache from lack of food. I simply rested my body in preparation for another day of practice, another day of tolerating the ever-present buzz of hunger.

Sunday evenings at Beth's were the worst. On the heels of a warm and almost-back-to-normal weekend at my house in New Jersey, the drop-offs were depressing. I carted my weekend bag inside, mournful over the departure of my mom and dad. In addition to the heartrending good-bye hugs, I faced the added anxiety on Sunday nights of anticipating dreaded Monday weigh-ins. I could only pray that the Saturday-night dinner with my family, a restaurant feast that inevitably included bread *and* dessert, didn't result in excessive weight gain. A half pound was tolerable. A full pound was punishable. To the floor I went, in my tiny bedroom, chasing the pounds away with hours of calisthenics before sleep.

# Chapter 18

I WAS NEARLY SIXTEEN YEARS OLD and an unknown on the senior circuit. I was preparing to compete in my first national competition as a Parkette and as a senior gymnast. I was required to requalify for the elite level in a zone meet, having missed the prior year entirely. Hosted by the Parkettes, I skated through zones without a struggle.

A new four-year Olympic cycle had been kicked off, and all of the 1984 U.S. team members had retired, making way for a new crop of girls. It was critical to begin résumé building with high rankings and international experience to ensure a spot on the 1988 team, a long three and half years away. I wished I had been born three years later, making me the perfect age of sixteen—rather than an over-the-hill nineteen—by the time the 1988 Olympics rolled around. My misfortunate birth year required me to stay in the top ranks for four competitive seasons, a pitiable circumstance, rarely achieved. Mary Lou had attained her top-ranking status just one year before the 1984

Olympics and retired soon after her landmark victory. In addition to sustaining high rankings over the course of four years, I would need to delay my post-gymnastics life for a year; I would graduate high school in 1987, requiring that I defer college until the subsequent year if I wanted to train through to the Olympics. Nearly four years of training, competing, and staying on top in the life of a gymnast is like decades. I lived in dog years, each day stretched out, each week of practice a struggle to be endured. I had a long road ahead of me, and this nationals, my first backed by the strength of an army, was critical to my future success.

I would be including all my newly learned tricks at nationals. I had the opportunity to make an impression on the judges not just with my performance but with the progress I'd made in the last year. They hadn't seen me since my botched showing at the U.S. Championships in Chicago. The goal was to make them think: if she can learn so much so fast, she has real potential. She could be a leader in U.S. gymnastics in a few years. I needed to convey that I was serious, no longer playing at an unremarkable club without genuine intentions of winning.

Gymnastics is not, and never has been, about who is objectively "the best." Politics loom large. Judges have favorite girls. Most judges have some club affiliation. They are hired to consult, to judge practice competitions. They develop an affinity for those girls in whom they've invested. There are also certain clubs that are known and accepted to be the best. The girls from these clubs are often given the benefit of the doubt. In 1985, Parkettes was considered one of the best clubs. SCATS, led by Don Peters, and Karolyi's, fronted by the famed Bela himself, were the best. But Parkettes was easily the third-ranking team.

If a girl herself is particularly accomplished, she is given tremendous leeway, no matter what club she currently hails from. She may have ascended the ranks with a top club and then chosen to go back to her original coach. By this time, she's already proven herself, so her name alone carries weight. Her mistakes and minor missteps can be forgiven. An unknown girl might perform a nearly flawless routine on beam. But a split-second leg bend during a tumbling series is debated by the judges. They don't know this girl. And though they can't agree unanimously that the leg was actually bent, they agree to take the full deduction. Another girl, a former champion, takes to the beam. An obvious bobble could rate anywhere between a one-tenth and a three-tenths deduction, depending on how generous the judges are feeling. The bobble's extremity is debatable. "It wasn't so bad, really," one judge might say. And they all agree. One tenth is all they need to take.

The argument goes: if a girl has struggled for years to earn her place in the top ten, or top six, or even top three, she deserves the benefit of the doubt. So what if she has a bad day? Isn't she better suited to represent the country in World Championships? The Olympics? Can't she be relied upon more than some unknown, who by chance performed better on a single given day? For this reason, it's difficult to break into the ranks. A newcomer has to be that much better than the well-known gymnast.

This nationals was my opportunity to prove myself and curry favor with the judges. Up until now, everything I'd accomplished had been without the forgiving generosity of a panel of judges in my corner. Lolo's wasn't considered a top club. She had no relationships with these arbiters of the sport. But now I had the power of the Parkettes on my side. I could walk in with confidence, knowing that the judges would assume I was pretty good, at least. And if I could parlay this effectively, I could begin to build goodwill of my own, based on *my* name and reputation, beyond Parkettes. This competition could be a turning point for me, the time to transform myself from an undistinguished girl amidst the throngs of national competitors to a United States gymnastics hopeful.

John was giddy with anticipation. While I'd competed admirably in the zone meet, we'd played it safe just to qualify. I had new tricks to unveil in nationals—a Tsuk full on vault, a Jaeger on bars, and two back handsprings to a layout on beam. Because he'd adopted me as "his girl" from my first day at Parkettes, he was personally invested in me. This meet was his chance as well as mine. He would have the opportunity to prove that his instincts were spot-on, that I was a talent worth staking claim to, that he was a head coach in his own right. We were in this together, praying for a top-twelve performance, exceeding everyone's expectations and qualifying for U.S. Championships, my first time out as a senior. The championships were the apex of national competition, the national champ crowned, runner-ups awarded national team membership. I had to make that meet. My future success and Olympic viability hinged on it.

John knew I was physically capable of delivering the performance we both envisioned. I'd developed unexpected strength in the last six months, strength I never knew I had. Strength I'd been certain didn't reside within me, if Gary Goodson was to be believed. No longer the Dough Girl, I was a lean, chiseled gymnast. This newfound physical strength allowed me to perform skills like a planche on the beam (the body lowered from a handstand into a horizontal position, parallel to the floor, held for three seconds). My quickness and athleticism had also been honed—I would perform a layout pike double back *and* a triple twist on the floor. And my grace and flexibility, always strengths, had been elevated. My pliability, a talent that allowed me to extend splits well beyond the required 180 degrees in leaps and handstands, made my compulsories stand out.

It was my nerves that had not been tested. John and the Strausses weren't sure how I'd hold up under the pressure. Would I be able to get through eight events—four compulsory, four optional—without a fall or major misstep? If I could keep the nerves at bay, focus on the task at hand, just let my body do what it had been doing in practice every day, I could prove myself a worthwhile investment for John. But the pressure of his "This is your chance!" attitude was unnerving. Lolo had always conveyed the perspective of "We're lucky to be here. Whatever you do in this meet, you're already a winner!" Not so at Parkettes. Qualifying was expected. It was achieving once qualified that set you apart. I set about this competition confident in my technical ability but burdened by the excessive nerves that came along with high expectations.

I marched into warm-ups with the strength of numbers behind me. There were more than ten of us in white and navy blue velour warm-up suits lined up on the competition floor for "The Star-Spangled Banner." My purple, green, and white leotard showed off my newly trim physique. Stomach muscles rippled beneath the light-colored, shiny fabric. My hair was done to Parkette perfection. Two French braids met in a ponytail pincurled into a lively spring. Precisely matched purple and green ribbons crowned the cheerful concoction.

My workouts had been going well. I could make ten beam routines in a row, five bar routines without a miss. I was on autopilot, my body able to perform these sets without my brain. But the new vault, the Tsuk full, still troubled me. I hadn't performed it without aid of some sort. I either threw it into the foam pit with a mat on top for a soft landing or with John spotting. It was unlike the Parkette coaches to allow me to throw a move in competition that I hadn't drilled thousands of times in practice on my own. But John was so anxious to have me show my stuff he figured it was worth taking the chance. It didn't need to be perfect. With the high starting value, even a big step on the landing would produce a competitive score, higher than what a lower-valued vault performed nearly perfectly would generate. And the adrenaline should get me through. On power events like vault and floor, nerves were less likely to interfere, less likely to co-opt precision. The extra surge of energy should enable me to make it to my feet on the other side of the horse, even if I couldn't do it in an everyday practice. I'd tried things for the first time solo in competition, with great success. I had done my first double back at an invitational in Buffalo. Lolo cheered my perfect landing, which took me to the floor finals and a second-place medal. I had nothing to lose and the odds were in my favor. I'd go for it.

After an admirable round of compulsories on the first day of competition, I started the second day with beam, my most improved event since joining Parkettes. Nonetheless, I hated starting with beam—everyone did. It was so easy to kick things off in the wrong direction with a fall. There was no chance to work through nerves with a power event to build confidence and expel shakiness. Beam required absolute, unwavering precision, a great challenge for a shaky first-time senior.

I surprised myself. I held the planche mount, nailed the tumbling series, and stuck my double-twist dismount. My confidence swelled, carrying me through my floor routine, the most relaxed event for me during competition. A new set, performed to Maynard Ferguson's version of "Nine to Five," was more fun than anything I'd flaunted in the past. It allowed me to showcase my dance ability while playing to the crowd. Two new tumbling runs were included. I'd performed the first—a layout pike—once before in competition with Lolo, but it was better now. My body remained outstretched longer, enhancing the difficulty, making it an entirely different and more respectable trick. The second run—a triple twist—was entirely new and added a notch of difficulty to get me to the coveted 10 start value. I stuck the first run, hammed it up through the dance moves, and bounced out of a slightly short landing on the triple twist (I got to about two and three quarters twists) as if I'd nailed it. Through my persuasive powers—a big smile and an enthusiastic flourish that included a back arched into a C and arms raised high behind my ears—I convinced the judges I'd actually made it three times around. They rewarded me with a 9.4. Halfway through the second day, I was poised to break in to the top half. I just had to make my final two routines.

Third came vault. Buoyed by the day's performance so far and firmly holding a spot in the top half, I knew a strong vault could put me solidly within the top third. This would mean going into championships with a good shot at making the national team. Despite the momentum, my nerves persisted—I didn't have the confidence of knowing I could perform this vault alone. I wasn't entirely sure my body knew what to do, even if stress took over and clouded my brain's ability to think clearly.

I stood at the end of the runway, preparing for my first go. John crouched near the horse, on the opposite side, prepared to catch me if something went awry. Competition rules permitted a coach near the equipment but not on the landing mat. It was intended to be a safety precaution, but if a coach wasn't on the mat underneath a girl when she was midair, it was unlikely that he could save her from a calamitous fall.

I took a deep breath as I fortified myself for the impending stunt. John nodded to me, pumped his fist in confidence as he signaled to the judge what vault I'd be performing. Judges are informed up front so that they know what to expect. It's the equivalent of a pool player announcing what ball in which pocket. A gymnast is evaluated against what she's committed to performing. There's no backing out halfway through, deciding against the full twist in the Tsuk. If my round-off onto the horse wasn't up to par and I thought I couldn't make the twist, I couldn't just fall back on a plain old tuck Tsukahara. That would result in a score of 0.

I rocked back on my heels and threw myself into a sprint toward the springboard. As I came into the horse, half-twist round-off entry, my hands weren't positioned correctly. I was too high, the weight on my hands not heavy enough, not allowing for a strong-enough push to hurl me through the air. But I didn't bail out. I stuck with it, as required by the competition rules—and more important, by John. Faintheartedness would show a timidity and lack of conviction I was not willing to demonstrate. I landed short, hands and feet at the same time. It stung. My ankle bent, the top of my foot nearly touching the shin. I shook it off. John patted me on the back. "Not bad," he said. "You've got it this time. You were high on the horse. Come into it a little lower."

As I walked back to my starting place at the end of the runway, my ankle wobbled. The bones shifted ever so slightly. I was concerned, but I put it out of my mind. It didn't seem normal, the common sting of a short landing, an everyday occurrence. It just didn't feel right. Bones felt unhinged. John saw me limping and he jogged toward me to make sure everything was okay. Arm around my shoulders, he leaned down to whisper in my ear, "You're okay, right? Let's do it this time. Then you're all done." I nodded, unwilling to disappoint. Not going again was simply not an option. It would be humiliating not to finish, having come so far. One more vault, then bars wouldn't be too hard to get through, even with a sprained ankle. I shook the foot, trying to wrest the pain, the sharpness of it clinging.

Again, I rocked back on my heels, hurling myself into a run. The ankle wiggled the whole way down the runway. I favored the other foot on the springboard. Again, I came in at too high of an angle on the horse. This time I barely completed the rotation, landing facedown, full twist only three quarters complete. I crashed into the mat, splayed on four bent limbs, lizardlike. *Crack*. I heard it. The ankle snapped. I could feel the bone come apart. Two unhinged bits of shin, rubbing together. John snatched me up off the mat, and I saluted the judge, on one foot, to indicate I was finished. If I hadn't, I would have received a 0 on the vault.

"It's broken," I said calmly, as he whisked me toward the bleachers.

"You don't know that." He looked down at my foot, already purple and bloated, the toes barely visible, the swelling had so quickly overtaken them. My mother rushed to me, crying. Her tears quelled my own. I felt the need to calm her.

"It's okay," I said.

"Mark, look at it. It's so swollen!" she wailed to my dad.

"Looks like it could be broken," said my dad. He fiddled with it, testing its stability. It wiggled in a way that a foot should not. "Yeah, it's broken," he pronounced in his doctor's manner. His diagnosis was mechanical, lacking a father's sympathy. Though now I can understand that he was purposefully keeping his tone light, not wanting to appear disappointed lest I see it as disappointment in me. And, in his own way, he was relating to his daughter, empathizing. My dad was an enthusiastic amateur athlete and proud veteran of broken bones, with fourteen to his name. We were cohorts now. Soldier athletes, committed to battle.

Disappointed and unsure what this would mean for the

rest of my season, I played it cool, too, mostly to keep my mother calm. I couldn't handle her tears. They seemed to signify hopelessness about my future with a simultaneous emphasis on just how crucial and important this day was. If she was desperate and discouraged, I must have really screwed up. As my mom descended from sniffles to sobs seeing her only daughter's ankle deform into an angry purple ball, I smiled. "I'll be okay." I wore my first broken bone as a badge of honor, signifying a rite of passage for the serious athlete. I did my one-touch on bars, logging a nominal score to show that I finished the meet. This allowed me to medal on floor and beam (not finishing would have taken me out of the competition and contention for any medals). It would also enable my coaches to petition me through to U.S. Championships, provided I couldn't recover in time for the next qualifying nationals.

While I was thwarted in the near term, I was also strangely encouraged. Before the nosedive on vault, I'd positioned myself for a strong finish. I'd let the judges know that I was a contender. Though it hadn't ended quite the way John or I had hoped, it was clear that if I could recover from this injury in time to make an appearance in championships, I'd solidify my reputation as a tough cookie, well worth John's investment.

A trainer bandaged me up for the trip home. Donna Strauss convinced my parents that we should avoid the local emergency room and wait until getting back to Allentown to see a doctor. I would need to see Dr. Dixon, the team's doctor, before we could make decisions about casts and treatment. Dr. Dixon was an orthopedist in cahoots with the Strausses. He issued prognoses only after consulting with Mrs. Strauss and fully understanding her plans for an athlete's progression. Once they colluded, they agreed upon the path for treatment that least interfered with training. While some might question his ethics in treating athlete patients, he was committed to enabling high performance in the short term. If he sometimes lacked the requisite concern for a girl's sustainable health, he understood that every gymnast wanted to be back in the gym as quickly as he would permit. Together Mrs. Strauss and Dr. Dixon always chose the path of minimal rest and recovery for the Parkette girls. Dr. Dixon was also the consulting doctor for the national cycling team, the training velodrome located in Allentown. Later he would be accused of experimenting with blood doping, a scandalous technique that involved flooding the cyclist's body with extra blood to increase his ability to take in oxygen. The procedure was crafted to elevate a cyclist's endurance without detectable and illegal performance-enhancing steroids. Not much was known about the possible long-term effects of blood doping on the cyclist's health. I would soon discover for myself that Dr. Dixon treated all of his patients with this same level of enthusiasm, creativity, and disregard.

Upon returning to Allentown, I visited Dr. Dixon with Mrs. Strauss by my side. An X-ray confirmed the break. They conspired, agreeing on the compromised solution that would allow me to heal sufficiently while returning to the gym in record time. A cast would be worn for ten days and ten days only. That would be enough time for the bone to fuse. Then, a removable air cast—essentially nothing more than a bandage— would be worn and practices resumed. And of course, physical therapy and conditioning would replace practice for those ten days in the cast. No opportunity to return home to New Jersey to be nursed back to health by my family.

This seemed perfectly acceptable to me, and I was relieved. If my parents were concerned about the course of treatment, they didn't express it to me. My enthusiasm must have quelled their doubts. While the foot looked unpleasant, I wasn't groaning in agony. In fact, I was smiling and hopeful. And a well-known orthopedist's official diagnosis ("a minor break") and prescription ("a week and a half off") was adequately confidence-building. Who were they to question his expertise? We nodded in ascension, and I set to work, maintaining my training without a blip in rigor.

Working out with slightly damaged body parts was normal at Parkettes. One girl, Tracy Butler, had been a top-six junior. She was about my age. She'd suffered a terrible elbow break the year she was transitioning from junior to senior. She missed a year of competition as she underwent multiple surgeries, first to pin the bones together, then to remove the metal adhesives. She was starting to practice again, but the arm never fully straightened. On bars, one arm was bent as she pushed herself into a handstand, her body precariously tilted. She always seemed on the brink of falling but somehow held fast. On beam, she danced, the right arm crooked at a forty-five-degree angle, an awkward chicken wing feigning grace. But it didn't stop her. She learned to compensate for the arm's weakness, the slanted way she had to perform tumbling moves. She simply found a way around her body's limitations. No one ever questioned whether she might cause permanent damage. Her parents were far away in Columbus, Ohio, not there to witness the agonizing and often scary ways she found to work around the damage to her arm. The coaches never worried whether she might lose use of the arm later in life. She persevered though afflicted and in pain. It's what was done.

It was with this attitude that I approached my recovery. The goal was that I'd be back to full practices in a month. In three months, I'd be ready for U.S. Championships; my coaches had secured a petition to put me through, given their influence and my placement in nationals before the fall. I would have to be ready. There was just no other option. If I missed the year-end meet, that would be two consecutive seasons forfeited. I'd have to wait an entire year to establish my ranking. I'd be seventeen years old and just beginning at an age when most girls were starting to consider retirement. The narrow window of opportunity in nationally competitive gymnastics was a brutal reality. This potential situation was unacceptable to me. I would compete in the U.S. Championships and qualify for the World Championship Team later in the year. I had my sights set.

My days began with physical therapy before school. The therapist, Bill, another employ of the Strausses, picked me up from Beth's at six-thirty and took me to his office, where he put me through range-of-movement exercises. Just because the ankle was immobilized didn't mean the rest of my leg needed to be. To hasten my recovery, it was crucial that I maintain flexibility in the other joints—the knee and the hip—as well as power in the surrounding muscles. I rode the bike for endurance and strength while he preached to me about his born-again Christian philosophy. We became friends. He informed me that, though he liked me, thought I was a nice girl, I'd be going to hell. I was Jewish and a nonbeliever. I needed to develop a "personal relationship with Jesus Christ" if I wanted to go to heaven. I laughed and kept pedaling.

When we were finished, Bill drove me to school. I hobbled between classes on my crutches before Mrs. Kuroda picked me up and dropped me at the gym. Despite the cast, I practiced bars. Since I was lopsided from the weight of the plaster, John spotted me through warm-up exercises. It was important that I didn't lose my "swing" in the next few weeks. With his spot, I even attempted more difficult tricks like free-hip handstands and giant swings. These didn't go well, the uneven weight unwieldy. We returned to the cast handstands, maintaining strength in the upper body without risking further injury. Then more conditioning. Endless sit-ups, push-ups, handstands held for what felt like hours. Leg lifts on bars with the added weight of the cast made my stomach muscles ironclad, the skin as thin as paper. Then, on to stretching and more stretching. I did splits with the front foot raised a foot off the floor, hips pressed to the ground, until my legs fell asleep.

Generally I went home early, before the other girls were finished practice. It was impossible to fill seven hours with one event and conditioning, so some accommodating parent, idling around the gym, would be nominated to give me a ride back to Beth's house. It was empty, as she was still coaching, her son with her at the gym, entertaining himself with the other female coaches' kids. There was a group of "gym kids" who played together while their mothers scolded other people's children. I was grateful for the time alone at Beth's. I could relax and pretend that I wasn't in someone else's house. I had free rein over the television. I could watch Phil Donahue empathize with cancer patients and the sexually abused. But with my crutches it was difficult to perform the simplest tasks, like getting a glass of water. So I gave the crutches up. I set them against the wall, tested the ankle, limped around the house fetching water and modest snacks for myself. I couldn't sit still, put my feet up, and enjoy the quiet. The loneliness of being away from home, injured and disappointed despite my optimistic disposition, required constant movement to keep from wallowing. At every commercial break I ventured into the kitchen, broken limb dragging behind, to grab a glass of water, a diet soda, a single apple slice.

My mom called frequently, worried about me all by myself. She hated to see me suffer. Though I hid my melancholy as best I could, it was during this time that we agreed that she would move to Allentown. My brother would move also, finally leaving Lolo's to join the Parkettes' brother team, Gymnastrum, following in my footsteps as he always did. The three of us would live in an apartment, and our family would keep the house in New Jersey for my dad to occupy all alone during the week. He needed to stay behind, tending to his pediatric practice, to fund all this training and travel to competitions.

I didn't think about the fact that Chris might miss his friends in Haddonfield and Philadelphia, that he might be disappointed not to graduate with his junior high class from The Philadelphia School, which he'd attended since first grade. I didn't care that he might be apprehensive about joining this new team where the coach, Larry Moyer, was known for shouting nonsensical, obscene epithets at his male gymnasts. I'd heard Larry yell at a young South American standout: "Licuergo! What the hell is the matter with you? I will shit on your chest and light it on fire if you don't turn it around!" These comments were so outrageous that the boys laughed, unlike the girls across the gym who, when berated, often cried. My brother had heard this talk from Larry on occasion when he visited the gym, viewing my workouts. Having to give up his civilized existence at Lolo's must have made him terrified and resentful of me. But I really never thought about it, didn't offer any words of empathy or a possible way out for him. I could have said, "This is my choice to be here. You guys don't have to be." But no. I wanted the Parkettes and my family.

I didn't think much about my dad's situation, either, that he might be lonely living all by himself in a sprawling ranch house intended for a family. On the weekends we would visit him, filling the house again, in the way he'd intended it to be inhabited when he purchased it for us in 1977. But during the week he was on his own. I didn't dream that he might be so lonesome he would seek companionship. I was sixteen and didn't understand these adult considerations. Nor did I reflect for a moment on my mom's feelings on the matter. It never entered my mind that she might feel she was putting her marriage at risk so that I could do gymnastics. I simply assumed parents were there to do their children's bidding, to allow them to pursue their talents to the culmination, no matter what the impact on the family. I know now that I would never leave my husband so that my child could pursue a goal, no matter how seemingly worthy. Our family being together, my commitment to my marriage, would take precedence. But my family was selfless and unquestioning in their commitment to me. And I didn't think about anyone but myself. I was undeniably relieved that I would no longer have to be without my mom, living in a stranger's house, while pursuing physically and emotionally strenuous training.

By the time I got the ankle cast off, my mom had rented an apartment across the street from Trexler Middle School, where my brother would enroll in seventh grade. The furnished apartment was a tan and plastic little box. The middle school was violent and scary compared with the pristine private school experience Chris had had up until now. On his first day, he was nearly attacked by the biggest and oldest eighth-grader in Allentown. When Chris accidentally tripped the student upon entering the building, he was challenged to a fight. My skinny brother—barely five feet tall and under a hundred pounds—was terror-stricken. He'd never been in a fight. Fights weren't had in cushy liberal private schools. Conflicts were resolved with open discussion. Not so in working-class Allentown. Fortunately, Chris was spontaneously rescued. A worthy opponent for this sixteen-year-old bloodthirsty aggressor stepped from the shadows and offered to fight the guy himself. He volunteered to stand in and take Chris's punches. This new friend, an eager fighter with a quick temper, was beaten to a pulp after school the next day. Chris was so distraught by the whole affair he never told my mom, so she never realized how truly awful this new school was. But at least now he had a friend, who came with a coterie of bigger, popular boys to serve as protectors.

Being reunited with most of my family encouraged me. My mom picked me up from school, drove me to practice, then physical therapy. She fixed dinners and packed lunches (which I no longer ate). We watched *Dynasty,* our favorite nighttime soap opera. I welcomed the return to seminormalcy; it bolstered my strength when the cast was removed and a withered leg was revealed.

Atrophy had shrunken my lower leg to half its former size. Though I was grateful that it saved me pounds on the scale, its function had diminished more than I would have thought possible in less than two weeks. Despite the avid therapy during my "time off," I would have a lot of rebuilding to do. The ankle was barely healed; it still felt wobbly. It was gangrenous green, still deformed with swelling. And it ached. It was the pain of cracked bones that would need to be endured in the months ahead. But that pain did not compare, it was ultimately bearable, in the face of losing something that was just barely beyond my grasp. At this recent nationals, I had almost secured a senior ranking. My fingertips had brushed near triumph, not even the thing itself. But I felt its fluttery seduction before it slipped away. Once I knew that thing existed, winning and all the accompanying applause and admiration, I launched myself toward it. My transformed self, the new solemn girl I'd become almost instantly upon moving into Beth's, the girl who was practiced at withstanding physical discomfort and any test of stamina, willed victory back.

# Chapter 19 THE NEXT FEW MONTHS OF TRAIN-

ing were merciless. Gymnastics is a punishing contact sport.
Much like football, the body is constantly colliding into for-
eign objects with brutal force. In football, it's another player
who crushes, bruises, breaks the athlete. In gymnastics, it's
the floor. Or the beam. Or any piece of unmoving, unforgiving equipment that meets the body on its descent through the
air from great heights. Each day I'd await the big crash. I
knew once I'd had my major fall—either a neck landing off
of the vault, a slipped hand on beam leading to a straddled
collision with the wood plank, a header on the floor exercise,
only one and three quarters of the way through my double
back—I would be safe for the rest of the day. No more crush-
ing blows or dangerous crash landings. One a day was all I
was good for. Fate knew not to deal me more than that.
Upon on surviving that first dangerous crash, I approached
the rest of my practice with reckless abandon.

My ankle hurt. It throbbed at the break and shot stabs of

vindictive pain up through the shin. I began to favor the opposite leg, the left, which caused shin splints, minor stress frac-
tures below the knee. Dr. Dixon prescribed choking horse
pills to relieve the discomfort. When I ran out of the prescription variety, I took five or six over-the-counter ibuprofen tab-
lets before practice. I'd need another three toward the middle
of my workout, just to get me through. Some days I'd feel confident that the relief from pain was due to healing and I'd skip
the medication. An hour into practice, I'd realize how well the
pills actually worked, numbing a pain so relentless that I was
barely able to walk, utterly unable to practice without them.

My weight became an obsessive struggle. Though I was sixteen and still not menstruating—my body fat not at the required
10 percent that prompts this transition into womanhood—I
viewed myself as fat. I was ninety-eight pounds, over five feet
tall. But the other Jen, my emaciated tour guide from my first
day, weighed eighty-seven pounds. I was beastly by comparison. And the weight so easily shed during my first months at
Parkettes fought to come back. Young bodies want to mature.
But I resisted. Unless the scale was moving downward, I was
failing. I gave up food before practice entirely. The simple
weight of a banana in my stomach could drive the scale up a
quarter of a pound. I'd save the banana or apple until after the
first weigh-in, then steal bites in between events, knowing that
I'd sweat the balance of the food off in water weight by the final scale confrontation at the end of practice. I restricted my
calorie count to five hundred on weekdays, less on Mondays,
when I was still battling the weekend's excesses. On Friday
nights and Saturdays I didn't count. I released myself from the
throes of constant calculations. But not without a price. Sundays were torture. I donned the "space suit"—silvery, non-
breathable sweats I'd been given one year as part of the USA
gymnastics uniform—and aerobicized for hours. To the tune

of Jane Fonda videotapes, I jumped and crunched, punched and kicked, for the better part of the afternoon. I denied myself food of any kind on Sundays, praying to make up for the meal I'd eaten Friday night. Or the bowl of ice cream I'd indulged in on Saturday.

At this point I had partners in crime. Several girls had moved into our tiny apartment, including Jen. She was welcomed into our little plastic box, along with Kristy and Alyssa, despite the cramped arrangements. My mom was happy to have the girls. It lightened my mood. The camaraderie of my teammates appeared as normal teenage friendship. In fact, it was centered on trading weight-loss tips and a cloaked but vicious competitiveness. The rivalry among us didn't necessarily come into play at the gym; we were all at different levels. Our potential for success varied and we accepted that. Jen and Kristy hoped to one day qualify for the elite level and make nationals. A top-ten ranking was unlikely if not unimaginable. Alyssa was my closest competitor in the gym, though generally a few skills and a few medals behind. The real competition among us girls was on the scale. And Jen was the clear winner, never crossing the ninety-pound mark. And I envied her. I envied her for her twenty-four-inch-waist jeans that hung loosely, for the way her chest sunk, exposing collarbones so clearly defined you could almost see the white. They popped above the neckline of her leotard, bragging. I looked at myself in comparison and saw a wide frame, covered in unsightly fat. A mere ten pounds heavier, I was convinced that standing next to her, I was repulsive. She was clean, free of earthly bodily needs—she didn't eat or even seem to want to. When she was at home with her family in New York, I poked around her things, looking for her secrets. I tried on her tiny jeans, hoping to squeeze into them, measuring my progress by the wrinkles in the thighs, the gap at the waistband.

One Sunday evening, when Jen had not yet returned from visiting her family for the weekend, I discovered a stash of laxatives in her dresser drawer. They were tucked beneath her socks, hidden away in a manila envelope. Huh, I thought. Is that how she did it? I replaced the foil-wrapped fake-chocolate squares, ensuring not a sock was out of place. But I remembered they were there. I considered the option when I felt particularly pudgy.

More and more, my mom, brother, and I stayed in Allentown over the weekends. My dad either stayed in New Jersey or came up to visit us. After a Saturday practice, I holed up in the apartment and committed myself to an afternoon of boredom-induced snacking (usually nothing more than a few teaspoons of peanut butter), which inevitably led to an evening of fidgety angst. Mere weeks after discovering Jen's secret, I found myself unable to allay my Saturday-evening anxieties any longer. If I adopted her methods, perhaps she wouldn't maintain her advantage over me. I had been playing with a handicap.

With my mother engrossed in fixing our evening meal (which I had no intentions of eating), I crept into Jen's room and swiped two Ex-lax embossed squares from her rainy-day reserves. The chalky fake chocolate was disgusting. I chewed with my front teeth, making every effort to prevent the paste from touching my tongue or mouth. The taste of it made me cringe and caused my stomach to lurch as the brown color and inevitable result brought to mind excrement. After the first time, it became a habit. Every Saturday after practice, I slipped into Jen's room to facilitate my purging. I couldn't bring myself to buy them on my own, but I couldn't forgo them either. I never took more than two at a time, and I never swallowed them on an evening preceding a workout. I was careful not to deplete her supply, to prevent suspicion. But there was always an ample cache. She replaced them herself when inventory got low.

Despite the rivalry, Jen and I were friends. We weren't vying for the same titles or medals. She would never beat me on the gymnastics floor; I would never beat her on the scale. Even if my new tactics brought me a bit closer to her weight, I would always carry at least eight or nine pounds more on my frame. This allowed a pure and binding friendship; we each got to win at something. Though I envied her leanness, I knew I'd never be as small. Though she envied my gymnastics ability, she knew she'd never get much past a low rank at nationals. We each had strengths. It seemed fair.

Oddly, the increasingly limited food intake and enhanced purging during this time fueled my energy. I learned to mistake the shaky lightheadedness of hunger as an energetic quality. I convinced myself that the hazy dizziness and speedy pulse were unlimited power with frenetic intensity. My consuming fear of the coaches also fueled my false energy. It drove me in a way that simple nourishment could not. Kryptonite strong, consistent fear masquerades as boundless liveliness, unmatched endurance and strength. I now craved the coaches' approval like an addict because I had experienced their wrath. Their castigations were to be avoided at any cost.

There were days when a simple wobble during a warm-up on beam could elicit a derisive comment, bringing on self-reproach and desperate shame. "Jesus, Sey. If you hadn't put on that extra half, maybe you'd be able to stay on the beam," Mrs. Strauss almost spit at me before walking away dismissively. Then there was the "I don't coach fat gymnasts!" line, screamed at the top of the lungs, reserved for the girls who gained more than a pound in a day. These gymnasts were threatened with removal from an upcoming competition or being banned from the gym entirely, the worst of all punishments for a girl who just wanted to practice, to improve.

The worst weight-related chiding, the most humiliating, was directed at young Lisa. A few years my junior, Lisa hadn't yet entered her first elite qualifier. She was barely ten and very tiny. But a muscular frame and morbidly obese parents made her the perfect prey for our coaches. After a minor weight gain one day, Mrs. Strauss took to the microphone, generally reserved for announcements during competitions. Lisa was on the floor exercise mat stretching. She knew it would be a rough day, but even she was surprised when Mrs. Strauss belted out over the sound system, "Hi, everyone! Look at Lisa there on the mat. She gained two pounds today. Lisa, at this rate you'll look like your mother in no time. Is that what you want?" *Click.* The microphone was turned off, and Mrs. Strauss left the office and returned to coaching. She ignored Lisa, who sat dumbfounded on the mat. Lisa's mother sat in the balcony, a regular watcher of practices, undoubtedly mortified. Astonishingly, nothing happened. Lisa may have cried a bit, out of embarrassment. Her mother did nothing. She didn't pull the girl out the door. She didn't even get up. All were willing to put up with these abuses if it meant a chance at winning.

Of course, there were non-weight-related rants and insults as well. Mr. Strauss was prone to throwing things when he was angry with one of his protégés. A metal folding chair was the biggest thing I ever saw him throw. This time a girl had landed short on a bar dismount. She ducked in time to miss the oncoming chair. Then she returned to the chalk dish, preparing for another go as he punctuated his tantrum with a disgusted wave of dismissal, a march to his office and a door slam. There were the more mundane and oft hurled epithets— "baby," "lazy," "C'mon! Is that all you can do?" "You don't even try!" "You never give me anything." "You're wasting my time." "You're wasting your time!" The list went on.

To a sixteen-year-old girl with a terrible and urgent need for approval, these words bruised. Verbal abuse heaped upon a girl, day after day, hour upon hour, forms a deep contusion, unhealing and indecent. During this time I was unraveling. As I raced toward my winning moment, I was fraying at the seams. My ankle was cracked, my shins were shattering, my hands were bloodied, my body was weak, and my mind was twisted. I was disappearing.

But I persevered through to the U.S. Championships, my first as a senior. Hungry and taped into a near cast at the ankle, I placed seventh all around and third on floor exercise. I went from unranked to a member of the core U.S. team. If 1985 had been an Olympic year, I would have qualified. I handily trampled my former rival, Angie, who still trained with Lolo. I'd come back from the broken ankle to secure my place in the national spotlight. John was vindicated in having bet on me. His muse had made good. I was happy but not surprised. I knew when I went to Parkettes that if I just followed instructions, I would succeed. Delightfully calm in my shining moment, I knew now that I could dig deeper than most. I accepted my medal on the podium, knowing this was just the beginning.

# Chapter 20

I WAS RANKED SEVENTH IN THE United States. It was the summer of 1985, and I had three years until the next Olympics, the landmark I paced myself against. My progress toward this goal had been steady. My recent surge in the rankings boosted my chances. The challenge would be maintaining momentum without burning out before it was time. I was walking a fine line, wearing myself thin. But all I could see was the goal and the narrowing distance between us.

Our cramped apartment had become too stifling for four girls, my brother, and my mother. With renewed commitment to our life in Allentown due to my success at the recent championships, my parents decided to make our move official. They sold their dream home in Haddonfield to buy a generic tract house with a swimming pool and plenty of room for gymnasts in training. My father would commute the two hours each way to and from Philadelphia for work, maintaining a schedule as brutal and draining as mine.

At this point, my parents completely gave up any semblance of their former lives for gymnastics. What had been tenuous was now completely gone. To accommodate three Parkette boarders, they bought a bigger house with less character and no earthy yard space. They let go of the house they'd been so proud of, that my dad had landscaped with his own hands. He gave up his backyard garden, where he had lovingly tended tomatoes, herbs, and zucchini. And my father, though he lived with us now, was rarely home. He worked long days, leaving at five in the morning to begin office hours at seven, arriving home at eight-thirty in the evening, after a taxing car ride. If he was too tired to make the drive home, he claimed that he slept on a cot in his office, though years later we would all learn that he had an affair with his office manager. He must have sought solace from the never-ending focus on the children, craving some adult attention for himself. Though marriages fall prey to strain and failure for many reasons, in this case, it was simple neglect. Everything was about the children, and not just the Sey kids but the other girls in the house as well. There were no signs of normal adult existence in our nondescript ranch house in Allentown. No dinner parties, no date nights for my parents. My mother's entire focus was usurped by us kids. My dad allowed her to pursue it, fulfilling his need for companionship elsewhere.

I spent at least seven hours a day at the gym, five days a week, sometimes six. Summers involved a five-hour morning practice, a short break, which consisted of viewing *General Hospital* and downing a few Diet Cokes, and then another three or so hours in the afternoon. My mom was the chauffeur. She drove us from the gym to home and back again. She washed our clothes and cooked food we did not eat. She adopted our eating habits, surviving on diet soda and losing ten pounds. I can only imagine that she must have found the solace in calorie counting that we had found. An obsession with not eating obscured more complex issues. Things like a struggling marriage and a miserable, though successful, daughter. She claimed that she couldn't bring herself to eat around us, but I believed it was a competition. Who could eat the least, who could lose the most, mom or daughter? She became one of us, a competitor with tunnel vision. She would be as responsible for my success as I was; she would enjoy the wins and mourn the losses with as much personal investment as I did.

I was reeling toward depression, out-of-control compulsive disordered eating and self-loathing. I was surly most days, disappointed with my performance during practice, pained by injuries, or anxious about my weight. All of the reasons I'd started gymnastics had disappeared. It was no longer fun. I was not developing a healthy body, mind, or sense of self-esteem. Now there was only winning. And my mother left me to my own devices, facilitating as needed, in the name of supporting my career. She left me to defend myself against the coaches who had only victory in mind.

In the fall, I began at a new high school with the other three girls in the house. Though Allentown was proud and supportive of their Parkettes—we were their national sports team, often featured in the local media—the public high school did not permit us to leave early for our training and wasn't tolerant of days missed for competitions. So we enrolled in Central Catholic High, home to large Irish and Italian Allentown families. The nuns accommodated our training schedules. We were permitted to leave at twelve-thirty, and no one cared how many days we missed as long as we kept our grades up. And they allowed us Jewish girls (Alyssa, one of our boarders, was also Jewish) to skip out on theology, which was really catechism. We were a band of puny outcasts in polyester green uniforms. There were twelve Parkettes who attended Central Catholic in

1985, my junior year. We were tormented by the other girls, their skirts hiked up a foot above the knees. They called us "Porkettes," threw things at us in the halls, whispered about our "having it easy" for getting to leave early. There was not a place for serious girls in a high school where most would not attend college, where many would marry upon graduating, become pregnant with their first child by the time we were midway through our freshman year at universities far beyond the Pennsylvania state line. They smoked and drank before school, taunting us from the parking lot, snorting at our prissiness. We kept our heads down, books hugged to our concave chests, and stuck together. We weren't popular, but we weren't alone.

Chris also started a new school. He was enrolled in the public high school, Allen, famously attended in the 1930s by Chrysler CEO Lee Iacocca (his portrait hung in the hallway). Now it was notoriously violent, replete with racially divided gangs. Because Chris's gym practices didn't begin until five o'clock, he was permitted a full school day, so Allen was the obvious choice. (Even with the enhanced intensity of training at Gymnastrum, the boys' training schedule never matched the girls'.) After his traumatic first day at Trexler Middle School, he'd become part of the in crowd. Though he was still the new kid and prohibitively scrawny, he was good-looking, drawing the attention of the local beauties, the ultimate entrée into popularity. I rarely spent time with him, other than to see him laughing on the other side of the gym when Larry shouted ludicrous obscenities. At home on the weekends, while I did aerobics and homework, I saw him through the prism of his girlfriends. There was a constant stream of beautiful girls knocking on the door, giggling in his room, hanging around the pool in bikinis. Barb, Angie, Daphne, and more. One was impossibly sexy. She worked at Victoria's Secret selling bras, naughty and unspeakable for a high school girl. They snuck in through the basement sliding door at all hours of the night, out through his window in the morning. I was socially and physically immature and had no experience with such dalliances. Chris was cool, and I envied him his social network and romantic entanglements.

As school began, workouts intensified. My recent climb in the ranks had qualified me for World Championship Trials in Minneapolis. With the competition nearing, I became more and more tired, eating less, training more. Longer hours, meant staying later in the gym, less sleep at night. A week before the meet, I was on balance beam. I spent a lot of time there, as my ankle still aggravated me. Beam was less punishing than floor or vault, so I often got a double helping and skipped tumbling. This allowed me to excel on the event that once challenged me and continued to challenge most. I felt more comfortable on this four-inch-wide high wire than I did walking the halls of Central Catholic.

My weight had become a point of conflict with my coaches. Robin pressured me to lose three pounds by the trials using "any means necessary." She suggested Vaseline, something she employed during her days as a gymnast. I'm not sure what she wanted me to do with it. Eat it? They threatened to pull me from the meet using the commonly hurled insult "I don't coach fat gymnasts." Ignoring Robin's suggestion, I put myself on an all-fruit-and-laxative diet.

By now I'd started buying laxatives on my own at the convenience store near our house. Jen's supply couldn't hold me any longer. I'd duck into the minimart after a run in the neighborhood, hiding the pills in the waistband of my sweat pants. I switched to the white pills to avoid having to taste the obscenely vile chocolate. I found something utterly perverse in trying to make the purging agents taste like a fattening treat that I was trying to expel from my body.

I was three days into my diet of apples, grapes, and Ex-lax. It was uncharacteristically hot for early September. Ninety-five-degree heat added to the strain on my already tired body. A bit dizzy and weak, I convinced myself this was nervous energy, even when my knees buckled every so often. I always caught myself before it was too late. I was on my fifth beam routine, having to "stick" ten in a row to move to the next event. I leaned into my final tumbling run, a round-off back hand-spring. My foot missed on the round-off, but momentum prevented me from stopping. I threw myself backward into the handspring, missing both hands and coming down on my head on the beam.

I crashed in a heap on the mat below the beam, semiconscious. I touched my head, saw blood on my fingers, and sank back into the mat. I wasn't sure what had happened, only that there was blood and throbbing in my hand.

Next thing I knew I was in Dr. Dixon's office with Mrs. Strauss. He told me that I'd cut my head, broken a few fingers. He offered that I probably had a concussion, though he couldn't be sure.

"No stitches in the head. She's got trials in a week," Donna ordered. He nodded. "She can't go with a shaved head in the front. It won't look right." He nodded again.

And I was on my way with taped-up fingers, a Band-Aid on my head, and a warning that I may experience some bruising around the eyes as the head bled downward into my face.

When I entered school the next day I looked perfectly normal. As the morning progressed, I felt pressure in my face and noticed kids looking at me, pointing and whispering. I excused myself from Sister Mary Theresa's Western civilization class to go to the bathroom. I was appalled when I looked in the mirror. Two deep-purple black eyes had formed. I looked like a boxer who'd lost a title fight. There was nothing I could do. I had no makeup to cover up, no sunglasses to obscure the bruises. I returned to class, head down, avoiding stares.

When I returned, Sister Mary Theresa informed me that the nurse wanted to see me in her office. Nervous, I complied. The nurse had me sit down. With the cajoling air of a parent confronting a child about repeated bad behavior, feigning concern to draw out an honest response, she asked, "Is there something you'd like to tell me?" I shook my head. What would I want to tell her? "Anything going on at home?" I furrowed my brow, utterly baffled. She touched her face at the cheekbone, indicating my eyes. An embarrassing realization shuddered through me.

I clarified as I touched my face with the bandaged fingers. "No. It happened at the gym. I fell off beam yesterday."

Relief transformed her face. All worry drained from her eyes, the tense pucker of her mouth relaxed instantly. "Of course," she said.

And it was all okay. My dad hadn't beaten me. The balance beam had.

When I relayed the story to my mom after school, we laughed. The suggestion that my parents would hurt me with physical violence was ludicrous to us both. And though she was alarmed by the bruises on my face, I assured her that they didn't hurt. And they didn't. Not compared with the broken ankle, shin splints, and broken fingers.

When I left for Minneapolis, the host city for the World Championship Trials, my eyes were a dark purple, the bruises edged in a sickly greenish yellow. I couldn't compete looking like this, of course. The meet would be televised. What would viewers think? They tuned in to watch pixies suited in patriotic red and blue bounce around the floor, smiling and throwing kisses. They didn't want to see Mike Tyson in a leotard.

A hairstylist, Cathy, usually came to important competitions with us. She French-braided our hair into ponytails, curling the loose ends into a perfect Shirley Temple coil, topping it all off with a shiny bow. For this meet, Cathy would have to do my makeup as well. She shopped especially for the trip, purchasing pancake stage makeup, as nothing else was heavy enough to cover the eggplant-colored contusions spread across my face.

For the premeet workout session I didn't conceal my bruises. I waltzed into the arena, exposed in all my purple glory. Finger bandaged, face bursting with injury, I approached my practice like any other. I was there to make the World Championship Team. Judges whispered. Some joked out loud, "John, you do that to her? Is that what happens when they miss a bar routine?" Coaches and judges who'd believed I had a chance to make the team now were not so sure.

On the first day of competition, compulsories (I was now known for these routines), my mother left before the meet even started. She was sickly and nervous. I didn't know she'd left. I was focused on the task at hand. And I nailed every routine. Mid- to high nines all around. I finished the day in second place. Just a hair out of first, behind Kelly Garrison, a veteran of international competition. Seventh had been one thing, good enough to get me here. But second? That was good enough to win. I was dumbfounded.

I found my father in the stands. "Where's Mom?" I asked. He winced. "What? Is she in the bathroom again?" I was familiar with her digestive struggles brought on by nerves.

"She's at the hotel. She left before you started. Diarrhea."

Ugh. It made me feel the same way I'd felt when I broke my ankle. When she couldn't stop crying and I felt I needed to comfort her. I was angry that she was so caught up in the whole thing, imbued it with such importance that it actually made her sick. She was supposed to keep some perspective, to tell me it would be okay no matter what.

I called her hotel to tell her the big news. "Hi, Mom."

"How did it go?" Her voice quivered.

"I'm in second."

Silence. "No, really," she urged. "What place are you in?"

"Mom, I'm in second. Really."

I had to put my dad on to convince her that I wasn't teasing. She thought I was trying to make her feel bad for missing the whole thing. With all the nerves, all the crying, did she not really consider that I could make the team? Why was she so incredulous? Of course my face was purple with bruises, but I was tough. Hadn't I already proven that? And if she didn't believe in my chances, then why didn't she take it all a little more lightly? Watch the meet with an air of "Whatever happens, happens"?

The second day presented a type of pressure I'd never experienced. The pressure of being on top, the pressure of expectation that necessitates the need not to choke. The air was solemn as we flocked to Cathy's room to have our hair done. I was first, as I needed the most work. We watched an old movie on TV, the kind that was on Sunday afternoons before the ubiquity of cable. It was called *Summer of '42,* and it was about a young man seeking out his first sexual encounter during a summer vacation in Nantucket. We were transfixed, grateful for the distraction, wistful for an experience we would never have. It took Cathy an hour to apply my makeup. The result was a face as white as the moon, practically glowing.

Shaky from lack of sleep—it was always impossible to sleep the night before a competition—and lack of food, not to mention nerves, I entered the arena perfectly coiffed. I felt confident, prepared to maintain my placement. I was performing some new skills with greater difficulty than my last national competition. My improvement on beam and bars was substantial, having spent many extra hours on these events with the pain in my ankle still troublesome. I must have looked a sight, pale-faced, fingers splinted, ankle trussed into a castlike encasement. Bars, my most nerve-racking event, would be first. The new release move—a Tkachev—was a complicated maneuver, new for female gymnasts at the time. For years it had been performed on the high bar by men, free to swing without the hindrance of a low bar. Women had to time the giant swing, piking the legs just in time to miss the low bar without losing momentum. At about three quarters of the way through the swing, when the body is outstretched, the back parallel to the floor, the legs kick downward and the hands let go of the bar. Counterintuitive but required, the hands release and the body switches direction, flipping back over the bar, turning 180 degrees so that the stomach now faces the floor. The hands reach out and catch the bar. Hopefully. When I missed this one, I missed it big, landing either on top of the bar or on my face on the floor. I performed it in practice all the time. But John was always behind the low bar ready to push me to a safe landing, facedown on the floor, if I sailed too far over the low bar. He would be there this time as well, but I was fearful. Not about my physical safety but about protecting my second-place position. If I missed, there would be no recovering. No World Championships.

I prepared to go, my future coming down to the next forty-five seconds. I exhaled deeply, discharging nerves. I raised my hand to the judge. Once I took the step into my mount, I was on autopilot. I entered a tunnel, not to see light until I came out at the other end. All I could do was go. I took the step and I was off. My swing felt good. I wound up for the Tkachev, released the bar, only vaguely aware of doing so. It was perfectly timed. I floated through the air, felt the bar and grabbed it. Done! I'd made it. John clapped victoriously behind me as I continued through with my routine, the worst of it, the riskiest piece, behind me. Thirty seconds later, after my dismount, I was standing on the blue mat below the bars, saluting the judge. I maintained my second-place position.

Beam was next. If I could make this routine, I was home free. I was trying out some difficult skills here as well. Two tumbling runs—double back handsprings into a layout flip and a round-off back handspring—and a double back dismount. I was armed with confidence. But on the balance beam, overconfidence can be a dangerous thing. Restraint was critical. The perfect dose of aggression—enough to "stick" the tough tricks—mediated by precision was required. The fact that I could consistently perform this routine in practice, ten perfect sets in a row, gave me courage. I attacked it, despite the splinted fingers, which made the tumbling a challenge. Beam didn't move as quickly as bars, the experience less tunnel-like. I was aware of things going on around me. I could hear cheers from the crowd, another girl's floor music. As I stepped down from a handstand, I noticed how my foot took up almost the entire width of the balance beam. As I prepared for my first tumbling series, feet together, I positioned one slightly behind the other to fit them on the beam. When I landed, without a wobble I felt my breathing steady. One down, three more big tricks to go. I felt the nerves and confidence simultaneously coursing through my head, my body. Every second on the beam was painstakingly accounted for, an entire lifetime of practices condensed into ninety seconds. The time moved slowly, deliberately. It was intensely lonely on the beam, more so than any other event. I felt exposed and vulnerable and agonizingly afraid.

But I did what I'd set out to do. Again, second event, the worst two now behind me. I got a 9.7 on beam. No one would beat it. Others would fall, as always happened on beam. The nemesis of most, the beam had become my friend. The final two events would be easy, all adrenaline, power, and performance. I made no mistakes. I finished tied for second (officially considered a third placement with two girls sharing the slot), just barely behind the winner. Just one year after having gone to Parkettes, one broken ankle, two black eyes, one eating disorder, untold boxes of laxatives, a few broken fingers, and splintered shins, I was the second-best gymnast in the country.

# Chapter 21

WORLD CHAMPIONSHIPS TRAINING camp was held at Parkettes in October 1985. All of the girls and the national coach, Don Peters, came to Allentown for two weeks so that we could train together before leaving for Montreal. As a team. Though I was at home, I didn't attend school for those two weeks. We trained all day. I was the second-ranked girl on the team, but there were others considered more worthy, girls who had logged major international experience.

There was Kelly Garrison, the veteran. Kelly had burst onto the scene in 1980, an unknown who blew the judges away with her grace and inventiveness. She was known for her courage—she had several outrageous skills named after her. There was Pam Bileck. She'd barely made the cut, but she'd been an Olympic Team member in 1984. That conferred a mythical status all its own. Despite her sizable weight gain since then (at least twenty pounds, usually death to a gymnast), the fact that Don was her personal coach gave her a considerable advantage over me in terms of status, respect, and ultimately, on-deck order for the meet.

Don had other girls on the team. He had Sabrina Mar, the "up-and-comer." She'd won the U.S. Championships earlier that year, a major feat given that it was her first competition as a senior. She had as little international experience as I did but was the coach's favorite. The U.S. judges liked her as well. Don also brought Marie Roethlisberger. Almost completely deaf, Marie was a miracle in the world of gymnastics, admired by all. Her father had been an Olympic gymnast, and her younger brother would go on to become the most decorated American male gymnast in history. And her disability, which profoundly affects balance, did not stop her.

Tracey Calore, former junior national champion and fellow Parkette, joined me on the squad. Yolande Mavity rounded out the team as the alternate, placing seventh at the trials. A "single" (she was alone, not joined by any of her club team-mates), Yo was consistent. She lumbered through, always placing in the top ten throughout the mid-1980s. A bigger girl, she came from a club that had been hailed as the best in the seventies. A decade later, it was no longer venerated. She carried the burden of extra weight and the name of a club past its prime.

We were the top seven who qualified to be official members of the 1985 World Championship Team. Six of us qualified to compete, though only five scores would be counted on each event. There were two additional alternates at the training camp, both from Don's club. He could decide as a result of performance during the two-week session that one of his alternates was more suited to take the stage in Montreal than one of the qualified girls. This authority was conferred upon him by the United States Gymnastics Federation. There were no governing rules. He was free to do whatever he thought best.

The pressure was salient, heavy, and thick in the chalky air of the Parkettes gym. The everyday anxiety with which I generally approached workouts was elevated to crisis level. I faced each practice as if it was a competition because despite my high ranking, I knew that I wasn't one of Don's favorites. He was a technician and I lacked proper technique; he thought that I was sloppy and unreliable. He would replace me in a second, if given a reason.

Within the first few days of camp, Yolande, Pam, and I were called into the Strausses' office. Don sat us down. We got the fat speech. The United States couldn't show up as the "fat team," he informed us. At this point, the United States was hoping for a fourth-place ranking internationally. The Berlin Wall had not yet fallen, and Eastern European countries still dominated the sport. None of the Western countries came close; their winning was still not as potentially life-altering as it was to those in eastern bloc countries, therefore their training was less exacting and oppressive. Though Mary Lou Retton had won the 1984 Olympics and led the United States to a second-place finish, the achievement was tainted by the fact that the Russians hadn't attended. And the Romanians nabbed the team title, their depth far greater than the United States'.

At this upcoming competition, fourth place for our relatively inexperienced team would be considered a victory. The Russians and Romanians would battle for first. The Chinese were a force vying for third, with the other Eastern Europeans—Hungarians, Bulgarians, East Germans—close at their heels. We would be proud to deliver a fourth-place finish. But Don insisted we wouldn't do it with the three of us being so fat. I looked around. Pam definitely had some weight to lose. She must have neared 115 pounds. Yolande was tall and big-boned, and while she didn't share Pam's lumpy appearance, I couldn't refute Don's accusation. She looked like she weighed about 120 pounds, elephantine in the world of gymnastics. By comparison, I was a puny 101. I'd finally tipped the hundred-pound mark, but still, I was flummoxed. How could I have ended up in this room with these girls? Pam had visible cellulite. Though she didn't actually jiggle, making the fat accusation debatable, Yolande had the solid appearance of a wrestler.

Clearly, Yo and I were on Don's list for replacement. And he simply couldn't have called this meeting without including Pam, even though she was one of his and would never be replaced. It would have appeared suspicious if the fattest girl wasn't there. He was clever.

I was devastated. A pound or two over my ideal weight, Mrs. Strauss was frustrated with me. She'd berated me during the weeks leading up to camp, without effect. I couldn't scrape the weight off my already lean body. And despite my own feelings of flabby grotesqueness, I knew that I was not in the same category as these girls. Don was aggressively trying to undermine my confidence, cause me to falter, thus giving him ostensible reason to replace me. And it was working. I was distracted during practice. All I could think about was how huge I must look, much bigger than I'd even considered, to be compared with Pam and Yo. I looked at them, disgusted. I looked like that? I needed to redouble my efforts. I stopped eating entirely.

Pam had other plans. Don told her she needed to lose thirteen pounds, approximately 10 percent of her body weight, if she was going to compete in the meet, which was two weeks away. Rather than curtail her eating, she gobbled laxatives. I used the pills to manage my weight, sneaking them on weekends to shed excess water or an exceptionally large meal. But Pam ate them like candy. I realized I hadn't effectively used this crutch thus far. I'd have to remember its efficaciousness when I got in a real bind. I had only two pounds to lose from the time Don sat me down until the competition. That had been relatively easy. I had done so before we left training camp.

Later I learned that Don did not, in fact, have an issue with my weight. I overheard a conversation between him and Mrs. Strauss that revealed that she'd asked him to include me in the discussion. She knew it would humiliate me to be compared to the other two, thus handily accomplishing her goal of getting me to drop the extra two pounds. He went along because it would arm him with ammunition to replace me if I couldn't meet weight. One vindictive move that ate away at my tenuous self-assuredness but, in their minds, killed two birds with one stone.

We arrived in Montreal led by Don to find that it would be an onerous task to bring home the fourth-place team medal. The Russians were like nothing I'd ever seen before. Oksana Omelianchik, a tiny first-time international competitor, took my breath away. Watching her practice her floor routine, set to a music track that mimicked birds chirping, I felt I had no place here. None of us did. She was beyond human, bounding through her tumbling series with back-to-back runs. She'd end her first pass with a double back, then rebound directly into a forward somersault, propelling herself into another run. No one had ever connected tumbling series like this before. She was inexhaustible, unrelenting in her spritely appeal. And she was not the Russians' only weapon. There was Elena Shushunova. Experienced, brawny, and serious, she was Oksana's opposite. These two were unbeatable. I decided after that first day of practice that I would be proud to get through the competition without a fall, to provide my team with consistency and steadiness, to bring our team to a top-six finish.

Two days before the meet, we embarked upon podium practice. In international competitions like Worlds and the

Olympics, the gymnasts compete on a podium, essentially a giant, wobbly ping-pong table. The equipment is staged atop the table, awaiting the gymnast. All others—the judges, coaches, teammates—remain below; no one is permitted on the podium but the competing athlete. This rickety setup was fine when it came to floor exercise and vault. It provided a bit more give on the landings, a touch more spring on the take-offs, which helped me, since my ankle was still not fully healed. But for bars and beam, the podium caused the equipment to shake and sway in a way that made staying on a bigger challenge than usual. The balance beam jiggled with every step. And when a girl on the floor exercise landed a tumbling run with a thud, the beam reacted, bucking with vengeance. The swaying of the bars changed the timing for swings and release moves. It was an adjustment. I couldn't believe we were forced to compete this way. It was like a tennis player accustomed to asphalt courts playing on grass at Wimbledon, having never practiced on the slippery surface.

We had two rehearsals on the podium to adapt, to reset our timing and steel ourselves against the wobbliness. It also gave us a chance to adjust to performing our routines without the coach nearby as a safety net; a pat on the back sent each girl up onto the podium to go it alone. If something went wrong, there would be no one there to catch us.

Other challenges rankled. Pam still had quite a few pounds to lose. We were all rooting for her because we needed her experience and her cool head. But we were concerned about her ability to lose the weight as well as the methods she employed in attempting to do so. Even if she made weight, would she be able to pull off a decent performance? I accompanied her to the drugstore at a mall in Montreal for a final round of laxatives. She was going to need to hole up for the next day or so, skipping podium practice, tethering herself to the bathroom.

Don must have known. She'd barely attended practice since we'd been in Canada, knowing her spot was only at risk if she didn't make weight. When she stepped on the scale at the final weigh-in, we all held our breath. And sure enough, exactly one hundred and two pounds. Goal weight. Thirteen pounds lost in less than two weeks. He congratulated her.

Now that Don conceded that the six girls who qualified would be the ones to compete, he finalized the order by event. And, just like it was back at my first international competition in Canada, I was first or second each time. (My Parkette-mate Tracey Calore didn't fare much better; we swapped positions from one event to the next.) Despite my high ranking coming into this meet, Don led with me in nearly every instance. Of course, it was all rationalized as "you're so consistent, you'll get us off to a good start!" and "it *is* your first major international competition." Nevermind that it was Sabrina's as well. She was *his* girl. I was nobody's. John and Mrs. Strauss accompanied me to Montreal but were not permitted on the training or competition floor. They had no influence.

I was undone, my confidence squelched more than it already had been with the weight talk and the Russian gymnasts. We all knew the likelihood of a team medal was slim. After watching the Eastern Europeans practice, I believe he relinquished aspirations of a team award and bet on as high of a finish as possible for his girls. The rest of us could go to hell. All that I'd done to enhance my stature had gotten me nowhere. I was nothing but the stepladder for Don's girls to climb up to the podium, the rabbit sent ahead to vet the low scores. If Sabrina and Pam made their routines, they might be able to secure a place in the individual all-around finals, guaranteeing a top-twenty finish, a mighty feat on an international stage.

I fought tears and set my sights squarely on simply doing

the best that I could with lousy positioning and no coaching. As we prepared to march out on the first day of competition, I was seized with nerves so extreme that I truly believed I wouldn't be able to go through with it. I desperately wanted Don to send in Yolande. I could barely walk, let alone perform a bar routine. The lump in my throat was so enormous I couldn't breathe through my mouth. I felt unrecognizable, my face pale and shiny, my eyes wet with gathering tears. Kelly, always the mother figure, sensed my desolation and quiet hysteria. She could see that my composure was shattered. And in an instant she turned it all around for me. With an encouraging hand on my shoulder and a friendly smile, she set me straight.

"You all right?" she said with her southern twang. "You can do this. Let's have some fun."

Her kindness gave me back myself. I *could* do this. I *had* to do this, for her. She was the top girl coming into this meet, and Don had screwed her as well. Despite her experience and ranking, he'd given her midrotation placements. She and I would get through this together.

Though my nerves relented, my performance on the first event was not promising. I missed a simple handstand on bars. Only five out of six scores were counted on each event, so everyone else had to make their routines to offset my mistake. And they did. I hadn't gotten us off to a good start, but now I had nothing to lose. I couldn't let Don be right about me.

My next event, beam, was commendable. I earned a 9.5, the third-highest score for our team, despite my first-up placement. Wobbly beam and all.

The fall on bars had brought me focus. I wouldn't go without a fight. Upon relinquishing the promise to stand out at this competition, I was free. Free to simply go for it. I wasn't going to win outright, so my sole focus became to prove Don wrong. My final two events that day were strong. My compulsory floor exercise earned another 9.5, and my vault was acceptable with a 9.3. No one missed a compulsory vault anyway. I made three out of four on the first day. Not ideal, but a nice recovery.

I was determined to make the next day even better. With a fall already under my belt, another seemed unlikely. During optionals, I'd throw caution to the wind and have fun. I would prove myself a force, not to be ejected by anyone. When the time came, Don laid a hand on my shoulder, sending me up onto the podium with a jab. "Get us off on the right foot to-day." He emphasized *today* obliquely but purposefully. I made my beam routine for a 9.3, the third-highest score for our team (the two higher were 9.325s, so I counted myself among the high scorers, with only a quarter of a tenth separating me from the top U.S. beam routines). Kelly, one of the most experienced members of our team, found herself on the ground mid-way through her beam routine. While I wasn't happy about her misstep, I felt vindicated in not being the worst performer. Don prompted it, not Kelly. More than anything, I didn't want him to be right about me. I didn't want his beliefs confirmed, validating my own worst suspicions about myself. That I had no place here in this meet or on the national team.

Floor and vault were going to be easy, another chance for redemption. And again, I brought respectable scores for my team with a 9.675 on vault and a 9.5 on floor. Even though I led the rotation, suggesting I should have been the lowest scorer, I was right in the middle of the pack.

We marched to our final event and we were unified, despite our coach's efforts to the contrary. I felt my pride restored. I deserved to be here, competing in this arena with world-class gymnasts. Rounding the corner into my last event, I felt more confident in my potential than I'd ever felt before. I would finish out this meet with no one in my corner. It was a step toward 1988. I was only beginning. I'd show them all—Rich Tobin for favoring Heather, Lolo for always believing Angie was truly better than I was, Bela for not choosing me, and Don for giving me a lousy spot in the rotation and calling me fat.

I prepared for my final routine on bars with my head held high. I chalked my hands and chewed my cheek and felt honored to be in this competition. My nerves finally gave way to pride. Nadia Comaneci, my idol from the 1976 Olympics, was judging bars. She was in her mid-twenties but aged beyond her years. Her hardened, lined, and overly made-up face made her look impenetrable, like what I thought a callous, unrelenting Communist would look like. Nonetheless, it was Nadia. I was buoyant. Things could not have turned out better for me here in Montreal.

I climbed the stairs to the podium, addressed the judge. My bar mount required a springboard, which would be pulled by Yolande before she hopped down, adhering to strict competition rules. Don would remain on the floor while I spun my set, no saving catches permitted if I should fall. I'd been practicing my new release move, the Tkachev, and performing it flawlessly in workouts. Don hadn't had to touch me once in the weeks we'd been training together. I wasn't concerned.

It was almost over, my first major international competition, and I felt triumphant. Determined to savor every moment of this last set, I exhaled and embarked upon my final routine. I wanted to remember it all. I took a few steps to the board, reaching for the high bar. Swung into a handstand. Swung into the release. Up up up. My body hovered. Not turning. Something was wrong. Terribly wrong. I released the bar too late, the timing of these bars different from what I was used to. The give was more extreme, the bounce more slothful. When I released, my body didn't spin. I wasn't flipping, positioning myself to grab the bar. I merely hovered, suspended above the bar interminably. Then dropping, precipitously. I was barely going to make it over the high bar at all. I skimmed it, my back grazing the fiberglass. Desperately, I reached through my legs, hoping that I could snag the bar despite the fact that my back, rather than my stomach, was parallel to the ground. My hands tapped the bar. I couldn't hold on; my weight was positioned too far away, my legs behind my head, straddled, rather than flipped back behind me. I was moving away from the bar instead of toward it. I sailed downward, still not flipping into a position conducive to a safe fall. Somehow, I managed to maneuver my body into a barely upright position, avoiding a head crash into the low bar. But I was still bringing my legs together as I hit the ground. My legs, closing from a straddled position, were moving upon impact. My feet splayed out to the side, all of my weight striking the right leg. Completely upright, no forward momentum that would allow me to absorb some of the fall with my hands, my stomach, even my face. All the weight, on that right leg. Knee bent awkwardly, horribly inward. I landed and I felt my body spin around that leg. I twisted, my upper body twirling like a top around my knee, foot unmoving. Finally, the spinning ended and I collapsed beside the springboard. The pain was unthinkably brutal, savage in its malevolence.

Where was my coach? My dad? A doctor? Anyone? Yolande screamed for someone to come and help. She was the only one who could see that this wasn't right. They were all on the floor beneath the podium, waiting for me to get up and finish my set. Who was going to come up here and save me? Who was going to make this stop, this wretched pain surging through me? They couldn't see that I hadn't fallen safely, that my leg was crooked and ugly, wrongly splayed. I tried to scream, but my stomach lurched. I grabbed the post that held the bars. No sound came.

John was the first to reach me. He must have been there in

seconds, but it felt like days. The trainer joined him. The world swirled around me. I was lying on the mat beneath the bars, when moments earlier I'd been flying. The trainer pulled on my leg trying to pop it back it in, convinced I'd dislocated my knee. Now I screamed. He had to stop. *Stop stop stop!* He kept pushing, bone against bone, grinding hatefully. The pain was odious, repugnant. He kept pushing and pushing. I grabbed the post that held the bars. I couldn't fight him. He thought if he could just put the joint back, I'd be okay. But he was wrong. He pushed and pushed and nothing moved.

Eventually, John and the trainer removed me from the podium so that the competition could continue. I was swept away in an ambulance, my dad by my side. The pain was extraordinary, vulgar. But even the pain didn't wash away the disappointment.

I wailed in agony, "What will I do? What will I do? I can't do anything but this. My knee! I'm done, and I can't do anything but this!" I sobbed with loss. How would I prove everyone wrong? How would I prove myself deserving?

My father cried and held my hand. "You can do anything you want to do. You're smart and beautiful, my baby. We'll go home, you'll finish high school, go to college."

Unhinged by fear and disappointment and rage and agonizing pain, I cried. I shrieked and moaned and bawled, mad with terror. And my dad held my hand and told me over and over that I could be anything I wanted to be. I was only sixteen. I could become whatever I wanted to become. He loved me. Mommy loved me. But we both knew all of this would be over. No more gymnastics. A new life would need to be discovered.

We chose Queen Elizabeth Hospital because it was English-speaking. Unfortunately, it required a forty-five-minute drive. Every pothole, every bounce, jostled the bones. The pain was jagged and filthy. It consumed, not neatly confined to a specific area but swallowing me whole. I was exhausted upon arrival. They sedated me immediately, easing the physical suffering, drowning out the anguish. I was wheeled into surgery. Hazily, I counted backward from one hundred, making it as far as ninety-seven. At four in the morning, I awoke to a full leg cast, hip to toe, and the "good news" that it was not my knee. The knee injury was death to a gymnast. The fabled anterior cruciate tear, which required endless reparative surgeries, was what I'd feared. Tammy Smith, a former Parkette, had been forced to retire from this injury.

I had broken my femur, one of the largest and strongest bones in the human body, nearly in two. The doctor had reset the bone while I was anesthetized, and luckily, there was no internal fixation (rods, screws, or plates) required to align and fuse the fracture. It was a supracondylar break, just above the knee joint, which would likely result in knee arthritis later in life. My coaches, who'd come to Montreal to watch the competition and to lend support, rallied around me.

"It's not your knee!" John cheered.

"It's only broken!" Mrs. Strauss rejoiced.

Hazy from the drugs, I felt relieved, hopeful. My parents, though crazed with worry and confusion, allowed themselves to be consoled by my enthusiasm. It seemed I might be able to return to the sport that put me in the hospital.

Gleeful, my coaches informed me that the U.S. team had placed sixth. We beat China and Hungary but were ousted by most of the eastern bloc. The Russians took the top spot, with their two bests—Oksana and Elena—tying for first in the all-around. Romania, East Germany, Bulgaria, and Czechoslovakia took places two through five. And while sixth wasn't what we'd hoped for, it still put us inside the noble ranks. It had earned us a team medal. This, in addition to the news about my injury, made me giddy. The doctors were confounded not only by my reaction—I was satisfied with a femur break—but by the injury itself. They had never seen a break such as this brought on by anything less than the force of a car accident. And I had managed it all on my own.

Everyone gathered around my bed in the recovery room and we celebrated. It seemed likely I'd do gymnastics again.

## Chapter 22

I ARRIVED HOME FROM MONTREAL in November after staying to watch my teammates compete in the individual finals. With a full leg cast, I sat in the audience and cheered Sabrina as she placed fourteenth in the all-around and sixth on vault. The U.S. men didn't fare quite as well. They secured a ninth-place team finish, and their highest individual placement was Tim Daggett, who was twenty-second in the all-around. Everyone signed my cast—even Bart Conner, 1984 Olympic gold medalist, who was a commentator at the meet. I was as encouraged as I could be, given the severity of the injury.

My father drove me directly from the Philadelphia airport to Dr. Dixon's office in Allentown. My parents had arrived separately at the airport on our departure, so they made the return haul from Philly to Allentown in separate cars. My mom, still sick with worry, fell asleep at the wheel, with my brother in the passenger seat. She skidded into the guardrail, awaking to the sound of scraping metal and squealing rubber. They both escaped without injuries, just another scare.

Mrs. Strauss escorted my father and me to Dr. Dixon's. She hovered as he examined the X-rays. He determined that a cast with a hinge at the knee would allow me to heal much faster and with less atrophy to the leg muscles, permitting a speedier return to the gym. He cut off my old-fashioned plaster cast and replaced it with a high-tech number. It was heavier due to the metal joint, but it allowed me to move the leg at the knee. At first this was a matter of degrees, a slight bend wreaking havoc on the broken bone. But over time, with hours of physical therapy each day, endless bending back and forth, I could flex it to almost forty-five degrees. This kept the knee limber and the quadriceps working, albeit modestly.

At the gym each day I did strength and conditioning exercises. Sit-ups, leg lifts, and splits for hours on end. I tried to ride the stationary bike, but the minimal bend in the cast and the jabbing pain in my leg didn't allow it. I took pain pills to sleep, but they gave me nightmares and panic attacks, so I stopped.

I refused to go to school. I sat propped up in the living room watching television in the mornings while doing my homework that the other girls brought me each day. I'd finish up around noon and head to the gym to practice with my teammates. Between the training camp, the competition, and the injury, I missed almost three months of school that year. It was remarkably easy to keep my grades up, preventing probing questions about when I might return to Central Catholic. Provided I maintained my grade point average, neither my mom nor the nuns urged me to go back to class. I claimed it was too hard to get around school with all the stairs. And it was. But the truth was I simply couldn't bear to hobble around my new school where I was already an outcast. I eventually went back after holiday break, limping along on my crutches, book bag draped awkwardly over one shoulder, tipping me precariously. When offered help from a stranger in the halls, I refused.

My mother's weeping was incessant. Seeing her daughter laid up in bed, leg bound in an unwieldy cast, was too much for her. As tough as I pretended to be out in the world—at physical therapy, at the gym, at school—I unleashed my emotional turmoil at home. I didn't let on that I was scared, but I was clear about being angry. I was spitting mad to be in this position, unsure about my future in gymnastics, the only thing I cared about, when I had only begun my international career. And I took it all out on my teary mom, who couldn't find the strength to tell me it was all going to be okay. She sat beside me, sniffling. And it made me want to punch her. "This is happening to me!" I wanted to shout. "Not you!" Instead I snipped at her every move. About my school uniform not being clean, about fixing a dinner with too much fat in it, about running out of Diet Coke. I hated that she cried and I hated that I needed her help to do everything. I couldn't learn to drive with the other girls with this clumsy cast on my leg, so she had to drive me everywhere. To therapy, to school, to the gym. I couldn't even go to the bathroom without her help at first. I was unable to lift the heavy cast to sit down on the toilet without her lifting my leg for me. The humiliation. Eventually we worked out a plan where she'd lift the leg, set it on the side of the tub, and leave me alone until I called for her. This ruled out heavy laxative use. So I was panicked about gaining weight, adding to my anxiety, rage, and self-pity. I couldn't bathe. She sponged me each night after practice, wiping the sweat from my back and forehead. I was a baby again, but she didn't coo and tell me how lovely everything was. How lovely I was. She just wept.

In January I was a month away from having my cast removed. I still weighed myself several times a day, subtracting about three pounds for the cast. One afternoon, I was reaching for my crutches as I hopped off the scale when I heard screams. They weren't coming from the practice floor. No one had fallen. The shrieking was coming from the office where the working moms had the television on to watch the *Challenger* space shuttle take off. And just over a minute into the flight from Cape Canaveral, Florida, the shuttle exploded. We all flocked to Mr. Strauss's office, where he turned on the TV. We watched in horror as the news programs played the live disaster over and over again, showing the cloud of smoke and fire and tumbling debris. Aghast, we didn't know what to make of this. In school we learned about the American space program; it was positioned as a tool in the American arsenal of superiority against the Russians, vaunted as more unnecessary proof that democracy trumped communism. All of that meant nothing to a bunch of teenagers training for nationals. But the picture of Christa McAuliffe, a thirty-seven-year-old mother of two, hoping to be the first teacher in space, chilled us. The coaches were speechless, riveted to the television, not requiring that we proceed with our workout. It was the only time we were ever allowed a break from practice. We watched together for over an hour, growing cold and sad, before returning to the workout floor. The day was lost, our athletic endeavors seeming trivial, inconsequential, in comparison with the loss of seven lives in the worst space disaster in history.

While the *Challenger* catastrophe jarred my perspective, I was not about to give up my fight to return to gymnastics. Though the import of real-life tragedy affected my outlook—my struggle now felt remarkably petty—I was heartened when Dr. Dixon recommended a switch to a lighter cast without a hinge. This new cast had measurable benefits. While I would not be able to flex the knee, I would be able to begin light bar practice. Never mind what would happen if I were to fall, leg still semibroken. I just wanted to get into the gym, to stop wasting precious time.

In February 1986, after three and a half months in all manner of casts, my leg was freed entirely. Dr. Dixon and the coaches agreed that fourteen weeks bound in plaster and fiberglass, two months shy of the recommended healing period, would be sufficient. I was about to turn seventeen, determined not to miss the approaching competition season. If I missed this year, 1987 would be even more pressure-filled, the year before the Olympics my only chance to prove my worthiness. I didn't argue and neither did my parents. My mom couldn't wait for me to get back into the gym full-time. If my anxiety about falling behind was eased, perhaps my mood would improve. My reentry into the gym would finally give her a break from being my full-time maid and all-around emotional whipping post.

When the cast was cut away, the look of my leg was appalling: withered to bone, even with all the therapy. My knee was the biggest part of my leg, swelling grossly below the thigh, which remained a greenish yellow, the color of pea soup. And the sores were ghastly. Something had itched horribly behind my knee in the last weeks of immobilization. I'd taken to shoving a wooden spoon into the cast to scratch. When that didn't reach, I unbent a hanger and rammed it down there. I felt the fragile skin on the back of my knee tearing as I jabbed the hanger deeper, but the relief from the itching was so great I didn't care.

The day had arrived. My leg was unleashed. And it looked nothing like my leg. The first step in coming back would be rebuilding the lost muscle in my right leg. Light jogging was a challenge, let alone tumbling and landing dismounts from bars. It would be a long road back, but I was prepared. The only obvious benefit of the atrophy was that I didn't gain a pound. The leg itself must have lost five, making up for the five I surely put on elsewhere. But as I began practicing, losing weight in my middle, the leg beefed up. I was a human seesaw.

In no time, I was bounding down the vault runway. I favored the left leg, to be sure. But I made it down the pathway. Like Tracy Butler with her bent arm dangling crooked and awkward at her side, I now had my own obvious war wound. I dragged my shriveled leg behind me while I tumbled on floor and attempted a sprint toward the vaulting horse. Flying through the air again made me ecstatic. Earthbound, I'd missed the soaring, the floating, the spinning weightlessness. The joy brought by each trick remastered was like learning it for the first time. I was happier in the gym now than I'd been since I was just starting at Lolo's. Every day was an accomplishment.

And the coaches were so encouraging. They withheld harsh words, knowing this injury had tested my fragile ego almost to the limit. They even ignored the extra pounds around my waist, the jiggle in my backside. They cheered me on, no one louder and more supportive than John. He was determined to usher me back. He'd bet on me, after all, on the first day I stepped into Parkettes. He wasn't about to let an injury get in the way of accomplishing his goal of training a champion.

My recovery was miraculous, thanks in no small part to John's determination. He was with me every minute, every day, of practice. The other girls were ignored completely, unless they were one of the Strausses' favorites. And in just a few months, I agreed with John that I was prepared to enter a national competition. There were a few minor maneuvers in the compulsories that I couldn't quite manage, dance moves that required squatting, bending the knee to the maximum while supporting my full weight. But I worked out a way to fake it, to move around the skill without skipping it entirely. And the judges would surely overlook these minor missteps. They all knew what had happened to me, after all. And I had finally earned "benefit of the doubt" status. I could've side-stepped nationals entirely. I would have been permitted to go right to the U.S. Championships, given my previous ranking and the fact that my very public injury engendered sympathy from the federation officials. But we decided I'd train for the national qualifier, test-drive the leg—and my nerves—at a meet before the big event.

My training shifted gears from relearning to preparing for a major competition. I went from performing single skills over and over to practicing routines, full sets requiring endurance and consistency. In all, the comeback wasn't nearly as horrible as I would've expected. I had stayed fit while in my cast. My upper body was stronger than ever, making bars easier. And my fear, the thing that had often held me back, had nearly evaporated. I'd experienced the most painful, horrendous injury I could have conjured. And I had survived it. Now I had nothing to fear.

I'd compete all the skills I'd thrown in worlds, even the Tkachev. That would be the most difficult thing to do again. Not because I was afraid of injury but because I'd lost all sense of the skill. Usually, in order to master a trick, the mind feels it in the body beforehand. We called it visualization. But it was more than picturing it. It was feeling exactly what it was like to perform the skill perfectly. It was like seeing with the whole body. When I was able to visualize a trick, I felt it in my toes, my chest, my fingertips. But I couldn't feel the Tkachev anymore;

the trick that nearly took me out of the sport was lost to me. When I tried to visualize it, I only saw myself missing it again, letting go too late, hovering stupidly above the bar. To throw it would be to go at it blindly, with no bodily awareness. John convinced me that was what I needed to do. Just get up there and go for it. Don't think about it. Don't try to picture it. Just wing it. Trust that my body knew what to do even if my head didn't.

So I did. Against all intuition, I closed my eyes and just stepped off the cliff. And I succeeded. The very first time I attacked that beastly release move, I nailed it. I cried. John cried. Everyone in the gym cried. My mom wept when she was told that I'd done it (she couldn't bear to watch from her perch in the gym's office). And I did it again and again and again. My sense of self was restored. Not only could I do gymnastics again, I could do the very trick that almost destroyed me. I was ready for competition.

Nationals were low-key. There were always two each year, both qualifiers for U.S. Championships. The first one was cutthroat, packed to capacity with girls vying for spots at the prestigious year-end ranking competition. The second was less well attended, as all the girls who'd already qualified stayed at home training for the big meet. Only the laggers entered, still hoping for a chance at championships. I showed up at the second nationals, in Denver, very quietly. A few heads turned. Everyone thought I was done for good. "Is she here to watch?" I could almost hear them say. When I took to the equipment during practice, I drew stares.

My compulsories were stronger than ever. Since the moves were less demanding on the body, I was able to practice them more, perfecting every minutiae. I competed well on the first day, placing in the top three. Going into optionals, I attacked the vault. Though I limped perceptibly, favoring my left leg, I tore down the runway seeking redemption. I landed my vault like an arrow shot straight into the ground. No steps. But the favoring of the left leg got me. I landed with a jolt, all my weight on the one leg. The mat gave way to the cement beneath. My left ankle crunched. I limped off the mat.

I calmly told John that it hurt. It swelled immediately, to bizarre proportions. I was so good at hurting myself I didn't even have to fall to do it. My landing had been flawless, the vault garnering a near-perfect score. And yet the foot was ruined. I decided not to go again, not to finish the meet. I'd earned the right to say when I was injured without being questioned. I was a girl who knew the difference between real pain and fleeting discomfort. Despite the lack of drama, this injury felt real. I was distraught, numb with frustration. Why couldn't I catch a break, go one meet without an injury?

I went to a nearby hospital for X-rays that revealed nothing. A clean bill of health was declared, but the ankle said otherwise. It throbbed, purple and fat, hot to the touch, the toes completely taken over by fluid in the foot. I limped home on crutches, again.

Dr. Dixon confirmed there was nothing wrong with the ankle. He was perplexed by its indigo shade and bulbous shape. "You're on the fence," he declared with a goofy, crooked grin. He meant, "I don't know what to tell you. It doesn't look right, but I can't find anything wrong."

I kept training. Without an official diagnosis, there was no reason not to. He shot me up with cortisone regularly; John taped the foot to castlike stiffness, retaping several times during each practice to maintain the solid bulwark. Each time the tape loosened, allowing the ankle to bend, he put on another layer, preventing any movement whatsoever.

The femur break—with all the hoopla accompanying a

severe injury experienced on an international stage—would prove nothing in comparison to this mysterious and undetermined ankle wound. But without an identifiable injury, I had no choice but to persevere, determined to see my way back to international competition.

# Chapter 23

MY GOAL AT 1986 U.S. CHAMPI-
onships: make the top eight to qualify for the first-ever Goodwill Games in Moscow. Media mogul Ted Turner had created
the games in response to the politics that divided the 1980
and 1984 Olympics, the intent being to unite athletes once
again, whatever divisions world politics prompted. My ankle
was a swollen, mysterious mess, still no diagnosis. But I was
confident. Armed with cortisone, painkillers, and loads of
athletic tape, I felt I could take on the world of United States
gymnastics, solidifying my place in the elite among the elite.
I was broken but tougher than ever; these girls didn't know
who they were dealing with. I could handle anything. John
understood this about me. Better than anyone, he knew how
mentally tough I'd become. He hoped for greatness.

Ten Parkettes were qualified. Three of us had a chance of
making the Goodwill Games. When I showed up at the arena
in Indianapolis for practice the day before the meet, all heads
turned; whispers filled the air. The word that I would be here

hadn't spread. Many still believed my injury at worlds was the end of my career. Most didn't know that I had been at nationals a month before. And those who did know had seen me get hurt again. They assumed that after two straight years of injuries, I would decide to call it quits. Yet here I was, happy and strong and proud, surrounded by my teammates, leading the pack of purple-and-white-suited Parkettes. I was leaner than ever, and my routines were jam-packed with difficulty.

There were new girls in this meet, contenders. Doe Yamashiro, one of Don Peters's gymnasts, was purported to be the one to beat. New on the national scene, she was graceful, strong, and technically perfect. Just the way Don liked them. He had spread the word about her for months before. And though she had no equity in the gymnastics world, he did. If Don said she was the best that U.S. gymnastics had to offer, then it was true. There was Hope Spivey, the West Virginia firecracker from my very own team, Bill's girl. This would be her first year as a senior. Whether she'd stand up under the pressure was questionable, but her naïve attitude suggested she might not even be aware that there *was* pressure, making it an easy task. And she certainly had the most difficulty of any girl in the meet. She beat me hands down in this area.

Of course, there were others, the usual collection of girls vying for the top spots. Sabrina Mar, the winner from the previous year. Yolande Mavity and Marie Roethlisberger, my World Championship teammates. Angie, who still proved to be worthy competition for me. The list went on.

The real stars in this competition were declared to be the juniors, the girls in the under-fourteen age bracket. Though they weren't able to compete in major international competitions yet, two of them—Kristie Phillips and Phoebe Mills— were Bela's girls, and they were promoted as the future of U.S. gymnastics. The rest of us seniors were being touted as "tweeners," almost over the hill but not quite, shining in between Olympic years. Sure to peter out before the next Games.

These younger girls were outstanding competitors. Their routines were packed with difficulty, rivaling that of the Russians. And though I would need to worry about them next year when they became seniors, I wasn't going to fret about the challenge they would present yet. I had the forty or so other senior gymnasts to contend with. Each had her own strengths, ranging from power to grace to simply being a fresh face on the scene. Mine was consistency. And my new fearlessness had served me well. Not only had I had relearned all my old tricks since my femur break, I had added some new ones. I would perform a double back beam dismount and multiple double backs on the floor exercise. And of course, I would tackle the Tkachev on bars, the skill that had cracked my thigh bone in Montreal. All of these skills narrowed the gap between me and Hope, as well as the other daredevils. I was confident that the discrepancy in difficulty that remained, I made up for and surpassed in grace, precision, and invariability. I simply wouldn't miss.

After the first day of competition, I was in second place, a repeat of the 1985 World Championship Trials compulsory performance. John and I were cautiously optimistic. Optionals would be the most challenging for me. The ankle made them painful, and I never knew when a landing would take me out for the day. Sometimes during practice one tumbling run could put me under for a full workout. And it didn't have to be a major fall. The left ankle was so fragile at this point that a perfect landing, of the ilk that put me in this situation in the first place, could send me to the trainer, foot plunged into a bucket of ice for the rest of the afternoon. And the femur injury was less than a year behind me. It generated pain as well, concentrated in the right knee, caused by scar tissue that grew as the bone healed. It made my knee creaky and jagged, the joint grinding with every movement. I had no leg to favor. But my general physical state was incidental, a mere inconvenience. We—John, the Strausses, my parents, and I—never questioned whether I should continue in pursuit of the dream of winning. Winning what? Anything. The vague sense that winning was the ultimate, the end-all-and-be-all, was our sustenance. It was more important than anything else. Health, happiness, the ability to walk in my not-too-distant adult future—these were distant runner-ups.

On the second day, I entered the arena focused and intrepid. My first event was balance beam, my best. I held an advantage over the others in this regard. No one's best event was beam. I didn't worry about falling. I concerned myself with how high a 9 I could score. And I was nearly perfect. A 9.6 put me in the lead off the bat. The announcer belted it out on the microphone as we marched from our first event to our second. "In first place, Jennifer Sey!" Never had those words been uttered on the national stage.

John was ecstatic. We high-fived, then huddled. He grabbed me by the shoulders, looked deep into my eyes. He didn't need to say a word. This could be it. All that we had worked for. If I could just hold on. I was undaunted. I marched onto the floor exercise mat beaming with confidence, shining with pride. I struck my initial pose and waited for the music to start. This instrumental version of "Nine to Five" was always a crowd-pleaser. For a split second, before the music sounded, I forgot my routine. A brief moment of panic struck and then I heard the first note and all was right. The moves flowed from my body without direction from my head. I danced to the corner with gusto. I was fearless. With a deep breath I set up for my first tumbling run. And I was off. Running, round-off, back handspring . . . I took to the

air for my double back, laid out to a pike position. A perfect
landing.

But the ankle jammed, shooting unexpectedly forceful pain
through my entire body. Tears shot to my eyes as I questioned
whether I could finish the routine. I considered walking off as
I danced tentatively through the next series. Caught between
melting into the ground, wallowing in the pain, and knowing
I could win, I chose to continue. But I knew I had to make
some adjustments. I could barely walk, let alone make it
through the planned moves, the double backs and double
twists. I went into the second run just hoping not to crumble. I
watered it down, performing something easy, less strenuous. I
don't even know what. The pain did not abate. I forced a
smile. I was two thirds of the way through. I could make it if I
just clenched my jaw and bore the wretched pain. Smiling
through tears, I continued, determined. The final challenge
would be the last tumbling run. I had to perform something
halfway decent or risk my first-place position. I decided on a
simple full twist, replacing the intended double back with
something completely unacceptable. I landed with a step and
struck my final pose. I burst into tears as I hopped off.

The judges, my parents, my teammates—none of them
knew what had happened. But John knew something was
wrong. He approached me, armed with his athletic tape, ready
to bandage me up so I could make it through the remaining
two events. Only he could tape it tight enough. The trainers
limply draped the tape around my ankle, more decoration
than support. He sat me down, undid the existing tape job,
which had torn during the first tumbling run, split up the
back near the Achilles tendon upon impact. He didn't even
entertain the idea that I might not finish. He got to taping and
talking. "One more tough one. That's it. Just get through vault
and you're home free. Bars will be easy." The Strausses and

other Parkettes gathered around me, whispering encouragement. I nodded, letting their enthusiasm wash over me. I was a boxer, cut and bleeding but not down for the count. I waited to hear my score, knowing it would not be stellar. 9.25. Not bad, considering I'd improvised, taking out a good portion of the difficulty. I was enjoying the benefit of the doubt from the judges. Incredibly, even with this marginal score, I maintained my lead. Others were falling all over the place. I saw loads of 8s. Sabrina Mar, the former national champion, logged an 8.5 on floor. The meet was still wide open.

John finished taping me up. The tape served a dual purpose—support and, because it was so tight, keeping the swelling at bay. I marched to the next event. The standard rotation order—vault, bars, beam, floor—was deemed an Olympic rotation. Every meet followed that set order. I'd started on beam, moved to floor. Next came vault. This would be tough. I could barely put weight on the left ankle now. I'd have to rely on the right leg, hardly in tip-top condition. But at this point, the formerly broken leg was better than the presently busted ankle. One vault was all I needed. Usually two were performed, but the rules of this competition dictated that the top score counted, not an average of the two vaults. I didn't take my warm-up. My damaged ankle couldn't stand more pounding than what was absolutely necessary. I saved my resolve, my limited pain allowance, for the real thing. For when it would mean something.

I stood at the end of the runway. Without my warm-up vault, I felt cold and tight. But I wasn't thinking about how to do this trick, *if* I could do this trick. All my energies were focused on surviving the throbbing in my left ankle. I hoped my body would just take over, performing the vault it knew how to do, while my mind focused on enduring the pain. John hovered near the horse at the other end. He would catch me if required. He would push me to the edge, then save me from total destruction. I addressed the judge, exhaled before launching myself into the next four seconds that could dictate my place in U.S. gymnastics. And I was off. I hopped down the runway. How I generated enough momentum to make it over the horse, let alone land my vault on the other side, I'll never be sure. I landed my layout Tsukahara on one foot, barely addressed the judge before John swept me up in his arms, ensuring I didn't put weight on the left foot. He asked for the score, impatient. A mid-9. I skipped the second go, betting on this respectable score to maintain my lead.

I was so close, I could touch it with my fingertips. I could win this competition, become the 1986 national champion. Made all the sweeter by the circumstances of the prior year. It would be the gymnastics comeback story of the decade: GYMNAST RECOVERS FROM CAREER-ENDING INJURY TO TAKE THE NATIONAL TITLE! I was surprisingly calm as John retaped the ankle. One vault had loosened the tape enough to make it useless. Bars would not put a lot of strain on the foot, but I had to jog into my mount and land my dismount from a great height, boomeranged from the high bar, at least twelve feet in the air. As if dropped from the height of a basketball net. John and I were solemnly undaunted. It was just us here in this arena. There were other Parkettes competing, but he was with me. His strength and belief in me were mine. We were each other's salvation. I would make him proud and accomplished, transformed into a head coach in his own right if he could get me through this meet and make me a champion.

The bar routine I would be performing was the one that had brought such agonizing defeat and injury just one year before. I took the warm-up, caught the Tkachev. I waited. I watched others prepare. I caught sight of those nipping at my heels, girls hungry for the championship. But none were as hungry, none were as desperate, as I was. Things moved slowly. Television orchestrated the pace, the meet recorded for network programming. One camera made it impossible for three girls, vying for first place, to go at the same time. I waited some more. The other two contenders—Hope and Doe—were on beam for their last event.

First was Hope. Beam was her weakest event. I tried not to watch, tried to focus on the task at hand. I chewed my lip, chalked my hands, glanced toward the balance beam, rechalked my hands. She was shaky as she prepared for her first big tumbling run. I turned away. I didn't want her to miss. I wanted to win fair and square, on my own merit, not because other girls fell. I focused on visualizing my bar set when I heard the gasps. I turned to look. There she stood. On the ground, beside the beam. I couldn't let it enter my mind, open up the possibility that I had wiggle room. Room for a mistake, a less-than-perfect performance. She finished up, and still, I had to wait. I watched the judges flash her score, an 8.8.

The cameras stayed near the balance beam, ready for Doe. This was one of her best events, but she was a novice in national competitions. She had a shaky start, a few stumbles. Ultimately, she, too, found herself on the ground after her major tumbling run. She looked stunned and disappointed. Her routine brought a disappointing 8.55.

It was my turn. I pressed my teeth into the blister inside my lip to jar myself from my daze. The prize was there for the taking. The gold medal was hanging right in front of me. I could feel the cold heft of it in my hand. But I still had to go. I had to make my routine before it would be handed to me. And then all uncertainty dissolved. Right before I addressed the judge, I knew I would win. With a conviction never before known to me, I knew I would be the next U.S. gymnastics champion. I might as well not have gone. I could have just walked over and taken the medal because it was mine. Then I was off, spinning through my set, the very routine that had crushed me in Montreal, with ease. I caught the Tkachev and flew through the rest. I smiled, actually smiled, while swinging my bar set. John stood by faithfully, under the bars, waiting for me to finish, ready to make a save. But it was done. No saves necessary. I saved myself.

I landed on one foot. He may have even caught me before I landed the dismount. The judges didn't care. They were on my side this time. And the tears came. His, mine, ours. The girls tackled me. The Strausses suffocated me. The joy was otherworldly. Finally, the misery and pain of the last year was matched with equal magnificence. The rapture of this moment made good on years of punishing work, misfortune, suffering. It was all worth it. Plainly, transcendently worth it. I could not walk to the trainer's table to have the tape removed from my ankle. I would limp on crutches to accept my gold medal. But it was the truest moment of my life. Pure and simple. Joy.

# Chapter 24

I SIGNED HUNDREDS OF AUTO-graphs while sitting with my foot in a bucket of ice. I ignored the whispers initiated by embittered coaches: "She didn't deserve it." "She only won because the others fell." "Kristie Phillips is the *real* champ." And after the splendor of the night subsided, I sat alone and I knew. I knew that what the upcoming year held for me would be unkind. It might prove insufferable.

In an instant, the glory of my win slipped away. I dawdled in the arena, gathering my things, accepting congratulations from my male champion counterpart, Tim Daggett. I wanted to draw the moment out because I knew it was already over. I'd barely had the time to be grateful. And though the scent of it lingered, it was gone. The joy, the exaltation. *Poof.* Winning disappeared, having gotten what it needed, no need for the winner anymore. Off to look for another.

I'd always been a fighter, a come-from-behind girl. Now that I was on top, the battle would be unwinnable. Now anything less than first place would be failure. I'd endured pain to win. But now that I'd won, what would be the point of sticking it out? The sad heaviness of it all set in immediately. Perhaps I'd peaked too soon, winning the championship two years before my ultimate goal. I'd been in such a hurry. Had I forgotten to pace myself? I simply was not sure I could manage another two years of training. Now that I'd finally made it to the top, the careening descent would require more robust courage than all the pain I had endured thus far.

Before wallowing in the emotional complexities of winning, I flew to my brother's first national competition. While I didn't usually attend his meets, this one was special, a milestone marking his entry into *real* competition. And I needed a rest, my ankle and leg having beaten me into temporary submission.

Chris was fourteen, skinny and nervous. I sat in the bleachers with my parents, but all eyes were on me, the new national champ. The little sisters of the boys in the meet flocked to me, asking questions about my injuries, wanting autographs. My brother was about to compete on the vault when an official announced, "Up on vault, Chris Sey, currently in twenty-seventh place. His sister, Jennifer Sey, the new national champion, is in the audience. Jennifer, could you stand up, please!"

It was horrible. Though I rarely thought of his feelings, I knew this had to hurt. The feeling sunk, stone heavy, in the pit of my stomach. This was *his* meet, *his* day, *his* first nationals. Sheepishly, I stood, raised my hand to the cheering crowd. I could see his dejection clear across the gym. No matter what he accomplished, he would always be second. In gymnastics, in our family. I won. He lost.

That summer I was part of a European world tour that kicked off with the Goodwill Games in Moscow, followed by exhibitions in Italy and France with their national teams. In one year's time, I had become the veteran, allowing me to secure top spots in the rotation for Moscow. We performed respectably as a team, garnering fourth place, a two-slot improvement from worlds the previous year. The remaining tour was all fun, no worries, no pressures. We saw the sights—the Eiffel Tower, the I. M. Pei pyramid at the Louvre—and swam in the sea off the island of Sardinia. I got drunk for the very first time, at a banquet in our honor. I flirted with a college boy on the U.S. men's team. Chuck Gerardo seemed impossibly sophisticated, a Stanford undergraduate with a biting sense of humor, and I found myself unable to resist his charms. He whisked me to the balcony off of his hotel room on Sardinia, spread a blanket across the cement, and laid me down gently. He was careful not to go too fast, keenly aware of my youthful inexperience, despite the fact that I was seventeen years old and about to enter my senior year of high school. After kissing for a while, I finally understood what this kissing stuff was all about, why people liked it so much. The way he ran his tongue smoothly across mine, our lips slippery and intermingled. I felt light, radiant. Luminous. I let him touch my nonexistent chest. I let him lay on top of me, fully clothed, pressing his weight down into me while we kissed. It seemed there was nothing better than feeling him, warm and heavy, on top of my slight frame. I didn't let it go any further—we remained clothed the entire time—but I was giddy. I thought about him, about the weight of him on top of me, for months after I returned home.

One girl didn't attend the European tour. Doe, Don's favorite, went home after the Moscow competition. Her ailing back prevented her from traveling to Italy and France, enjoying the spoils of our accomplishments. Though I knew her back ached, I thought Don used it as a legitimate excuse to send her home. He wanted to shield her from the world so that he could keep her for himself. He was clearly enamored of her; he admired her promise, youth, and tenacity. It was rumored that something was going on between Doe and Don, something more than a coach/gymnast relationship. That perhaps there were improprieties. A quiet girl, Doe kept to herself or spent time with Don during most of our stay in Russia, adding weight to the rumors. Even Mrs. Strauss conceded that it might be true. It got to the point where we all joked about it. "Where's Doe?" one girl would say, and we would all fall into a pile in fits of laughter. Yet no one intervened. Nobody asked Don, "What's going on here?" Everyone just let it happen.

After a month on tour, I returned home to Allentown, a champion. I'd gained weight, eating delicious Italian food, freed from the pressures of twice-daily weigh-ins. It must have been really noticeable. An older man who used to enjoy watching our practices commented, "Wow. You've really gotten heavy. What are you up to, 110?" No. I weighed 107. But how did he get so close? Did he look at the weight charts? He seemed angry and disappointed, as if I'd let him down. Twisted man. I had enough people on me about the six pounds I'd gained. I didn't need a near-blind, feeble spectator chiming in as well.

Once I was back in Allentown, hazy gloom and angry frustration set in. I had two years to maintain this intensity of training, two years of enduring this constant hunger and physical pain. More X-rays of my ankle showed nothing. The foot remained distorted, but all of the doctors—Dr. Dixon and other specialists—insisted that it was fine. Worst of all, I was a senior in high school. The two years would mean delaying college. I'd known this all along, but somehow now it felt unthinkable. I wanted out.

Depression set in, heavy and suffocating. It obscured my

vision and blocked my abilities. Simple moves, things I had been performing for years, became impossible for me. I got the "spins," not uncommon among seasoned gymnasts. I had no sense of myself in the air. I'd become lost midtrick. Undone, I'd bail out midair. A recipe for injury. I became so afraid after any number of scary crashes that I refused to try anything. I was so overweight, I couldn't perform tricks that nine-years-olds had mastered. My coaches were incensed. Practices were harrowing. John, in particular, felt betrayed. After all we had battled together, he raged against my giving up now. "You're not even trying! What the hell is the matter with you!" he screamed during a particularly pointless and frustrating bar practice.

Mrs. Strauss couldn't help but chime in. Her gym's reputation was at stake. "Jesus, Sey! You're throwing it all away. No wonder you can't do anything. You're fat!"

I sat dejected beside the bars, chewing my mouth, debating my options. Get back up, fall again, walk out. None of these were appealing. My mind raced over the turmoil of the past year. How could I explain that it had left me? The power and certainty and intuitive sense of how to do the seemingly impossible—*poof*. Gone. The audacity to try—also gone. I was clumsy and lethargic. I landed on my face time and time again. Rug burns under my nose scabbed over into a bloody clump, landing me in the school nurse's office again. I felt utterly hopeless. I knew I should want to continue. I'd been on autopilot for so long—I did what my coaches told me, I ignored doubt and injury. And now, out of nowhere, I questioned. Why do this anymore? Why continue? My body pained me all the time. The continuous hurt was draining. I was tired, all my energy wasted in battling injury. The comeback had sapped me, leaving me shell-shocked and exhausted. I limped through school, dreaded practice.

My weight became an all-out battle. The laxative use turned to abuse. I gulped pills, running through at least one package of twenty-four each week. I had to rotate my purchasing, walking from grocery store to drugstore, so as to avoid suspicion on the part of the clerks. I hoarded packages to ensure I never ran out. If I found myself in the mall with my housemates, I'd slip off to the CVS pharmacy, sliding a box of Ex-lax in with my Diet Coke, hoping the clerk wouldn't put two and two together. A skinny girl buying diet soda and laxatives. Or I'd run to the grocery store when my mom ran out of milk. I'd offer enthusiastically, taking her money to stock up on pills. She thought I just wanted to practice driving, only recently having secured my license. I built tolerance due to overuse. My former dosage did not work at all. I had to take six, seven, eight pills to prompt expulsion and potential temporary weight loss. And still, I gained weight. I hovered at around 105, sometimes as high as 107 pounds. In my mind, this number, well over the evil 100-pound mark, was disgusting. Amongst the 80-pound sprites who twirled around me I was a beast. My seventeen-year-old body was fighting to fill out. Though my body-fat percentage was still low—around 3 percent, well below the 10 to 12 required to menstruate—I was convinced that I was obese.

"I can see the fat on you!" Mrs. Strauss howled. "Can't you see yourself? After all this. All we've done. You're gonna give it all away. You're nothing!"

John had taken up coaching a younger, happier girl on another set of bars. Mrs. Strauss looked as if she wanted to kick me, but she simply walked away muttering obscenities. I fought tears as I rechalked my hands, pondering my next move. I believed the things she said. I believed I deserved their abuse and abandonment. In that moment, I believed I was nothing.

# Chapter 25

A FEW THINGS BRIGHTENED MY mood, albeit briefly, during the 1986–1987 school year, my senior year. I was honored with the Olympic Committee's Athlete of the Year award for gymnastics. Mrs. Strauss kept it a secret from me when we flew to St. Louis for a supposed clinic. She was vague about the details, how I needed to prepare. When we gathered for a celebratory banquet in the hotel's ballroom, I was confused. When an Olympic Committee member called me to the podium after citing my accomplishments, I was aghast, completely choked up. It brought back a semblance of the pride I'd felt months earlier upon winning.

I also snagged a boyfriend during my senior year. Mike was a junior with a reputation for being a bad boy. I didn't really know what that meant, but it sounded good. He was cute and nice to me and enamored of my little-girl's body. What I saw as bulky and repulsive, he found delicate and sweetly virginal. He was also taken with my dedication and my stature in our modest town. I was famous in his eyes. The Allentown *Morning Call* and *The Philadelphia Inquirer* featured stories about me on a regular basis. Sometimes, before a big meet, I was on the local five o'clock news as "local girl on the road to gold." I'd even appeared on *Good Morning America* after my win at the U.S. Championships.

The relationship started innocently. He liked Alyssa, one of the girls who lived at our house and also attended Central Catholic High. One Friday night he came by to pick her up for a date they'd arranged in school that day. But she decided to go home for the weekend instead, and she asked me to let Mike know that they'd have to reschedule. Shy in the ways of dating, she was too embarrassed to call him herself and cancel. When he honked the car horn while parked at the curb outside my house, I ran out to tell him that she'd gone home to see her parents in New Jersey.

"Why don't you come with me, then?"

"Me? I can't," I said.

"C'mon," he urged.

I pondered his offer. "Okay," I said, surprising myself. I ran inside to tell my mom I was going out. Because I seemed happy for the first time in months, she didn't question where.

I pulled on my cutest jeans, the ones with zippers at the ankles, and ran outside. I hopped into the car, having no idea what the night had in store. Four hours later, with ice cream (him), talking (me), and miniature golf under our belts, I was in like. He was, too. When he dropped me off, he turned to me and said, "What are we going to do?" About Alyssa, he meant. I shrugged, enamored of the adultness of the situation. It was illicit. He was supposed to be with her, but he liked me and I liked him. And she was my friend. It was all so delightfully adulterous and grown-up. We agreed not to say anything, to see what happened.

But at school, we couldn't ignore each other. He lingered by my locker, escorted me to class. Alyssa knew immediately. She feigned anger but ultimately released him, freeing me to embark upon my first real relationship. Mike kissed me in the halls at school, forcing the nuns to part us as the bell rang. We spent entire weekends together. We went to Friday-night high school football games, Saturday-night parties that I had never been invited to before. These usually took place in the parking lot behind school, "the pits." Kids got drunk on beer and whiskey while Mike propped himself on his car bumper with his arm around my shoulder. He nursed a beer, knowing the drinking made me uncomfortable. Sundays were spent at his house, lingering in front of the television, me pretending to watch the sports match-ups.

Mike was rumored to be a heavy drinker and sometime drug user. I never saw any bad behavior on his part, though his breath often smelled sweetly antiseptic in the mornings when I kissed him before homeroom. (I later recognized the smell as cinnamon gum obscuring the lingering scent of whiskey.) He always appeared quaintly sober in front of me. In my mind, if the gist of the rumors were to be believed, his sobriety was a testament to how much he really liked me.

While we pretended to watch Sunday football games, we were really waiting for his parents to leave so we could fool around. When they left for the grocery store to collect the ingredients for a lavish Italian Sunday dinner, Mike came at me. And I didn't mind. He pushed it as far as he could, and I let him go as far as I felt safe. In Sardinia, Chuck had warmed me up to the idea of sex. Though I remained as passive with Mike as I had been with Chuck, I let him slide his hand inside my underwear, my breath catching every time he did. If we knew his parents would be gone a long time, I would let him remove all of my clothes and then his own. The warmth of his body, heavy on top of mine, felt like safety. And love. It often brought tears to my eyes, a fact that confounded him. Though I was tempted by the prospect of sex, it was still a line I was not willing to cross, tied as I was to the idea of myself as a girl, not a woman. Ultimately, I guarded my virgin status, much to Mike's dismay and frustration.

"You're going to give me blue balls," he'd whine. I'd crack a sheepish smile, averting my eyes and exaggerating my innocence, feeling proud that I could inflict such a malady.

Upon his parents' return, our clothes were disheveled, our faces red from friction. Of course they knew, but they liked me. I was recognized in the local community for my accomplishments. I got straight A's. They believed me to be a good influence on their son, who'd often been in trouble in school. Admiring me for my quiet dedication, his parents welcomed me in their home, even if I fooled around with their son while they made a trip to the market. They didn't care if I never did gymnastics again.

I loved being with Mike. We had fun even when we weren't fooling around. We went sledding in the winter, something I hadn't entertained since I was a small child, too fearful of injuries that might result from careening down an icy hill. We went to the movies and held hands in the back row. He took me out to dinner to adult places like the King George Inn, Allentown's most sophisticated restaurant. And we talked. He listened to me go on about my struggles in the gym.

"Just quit," he would always say, bewildered as to why this was even a difficult decision. He always did exactly what he wanted to do, never worried about consequences or disappointing his parents. And, he figured, I'd already accomplished so much. It seemed an obviously easy choice. Leave while still on top. Move on.

"I can't," I'd say. Unable to really explain why quitting was unfathomable, I'd lay my head on his shoulder and cry. He'd wipe my tears as I dreaded the next day's practice and weigh-in. Though I never said it, I thought I loved him. He told me that he loved me all the time, an assertion that made me decidedly uncomfortable. Though he had wooed me, I felt undeserving of his affections, too childish to be the object of anyone's mature and seemingly unconditional love.

My brother, now a sophomore at Allen High, didn't like Mike. He made it very clear that he did not approve of my relationship with this ne'er-do-well. Chris probably didn't like me very much either, having sat by for most of his life while I consumed the attentions of our parents. His distaste for Mike and resentment toward me compelled him to interfere. He was intent on thwarting me in the area of life where he had always been superior. I could have all the medals and championships, but I wasn't going to have more fun or romance.

Chris had a lot of friends. On the weekends, he traveled in a pack of six guys, all cute and cocky, the kings of Allentown. Most of them were from well-to-do families, and they attended nearby prep schools after graduating from Trexler Middle School. Their families considered them far too special to attend the blue-collar, low-class Allen High. They were preppy, chiseled, and tan, beautiful high school boy specimens moving effortlessly through their teenage years. They seemed to actually glow, blessed and enviable in their absolute certainty of their place in the world. Chris continued to have a bevy of girlfriends, a constant stream of bikini-clad young women with tiny waists, developed busts, and cigarettes dangling from their pouty lips.

Because my brother was so thoroughly entrenched in the Allentown high school scene, he heard rumors about Mike that I, as an outsider, was not privy to. Chris swore to me that Mike was still a drunk, stumbling and fighting his way through parties when I chose to stay home. When I refused to listen, he told me that Mike cheated, getting blow jobs from slutty girls in his car when I was away at competitions. Chris took on the protective air of a big brother in this situation because, even though he was younger, he was more experienced in the ways of dating. And though I believe he truly wanted to protect me, I think he also derived a spiteful thrill from seeing my heart wrenched. He'd been disappointed so many times because of me. He was yanked from two gymnastics teams where he had friends and coaches who he liked. He was pulled from the elementary school that he loved. He had to move to Allentown and face deviant eighth-grade sadists who wanted to beat him to a pulp on a regular basis. He must have felt that I'd ruined his life. So when he told me about Mike's indiscretions, under the guise of shielding me from indignities, he took glee in doing so, though it was barely detectable. He expertly hid his satisfaction, revealing only the caring exterior of a loving brother. He told me these horrible things but "forgot" to tell me when Mike called the house, giving his true intentions away. Intent on asserting his authority in the house, and finally exerting some control in the family, my brother sabotaged the relationship.

What Chris wasn't aware of was that I was willing to let him have the spotlight. He did not have to interfere in my love life to feel powerful. I would have been happy to have him take over the family's focus so that I could be left alone to sit quietly on the couch, holding hands with Mike. Though I was afraid to let go of all that I'd worked for, afraid of regret and disappointing my parents and coaches, I was more content with Mike than I'd felt since I was a small child just starting in the gym. Mike was my only ally.

My parents weren't paying attention to the obvious signs of depression and self-abuse. They didn't seem to notice the lethargy, inability to sleep, excessive laxative use, and near-starvation diet. They ignored any fact of my life that was not related to the gym. Not once did they ask me about Mike, happy to pretend that I didn't have a boyfriend and that I wasn't growing up and away from the gym. His calls, his presence, and my absence on Saturday nights were ignored. They never posed a single question about our relationship. Not one "Do you love him?" or "Does he treat you nicely?" or "Are you having sex?" Nothing. There was no discussion at all about the matter.

All that mattered was that I was the national champion with two more years to go before the Olympics. And Chris, though years ahead of me in social experience, was a struggling gymnast. In this, he envied my position and simply could not understand why I would want to give up now. It seemed to him that failing to continue with gymnastics would be squandering my good fortune and star position in the family. To forsake the crowning glory—an Olympic Team spot—was incomprehensible.

Ultimately, I learned that the things Chris told me about Mike were true. The drinking and drug use were excusable, but I found the cheating too embarrassing to endure. Each Saturday night, after dropping me off at home at eleven o'clock, he returned to the party we had just left together to find a willing girl. He would take her to his car where they would have sex or she would kneel down on the floor while he leaned back and closed his eyes, letting her alleviate the blue balls I'd so cruelly inflicted. I broke up with him even though I believed I still loved him. He didn't ask much of me other than to be a normal high school girl. I was willing to let him drink and cavort. I denied him sex, so it seemed only fair. But in the end, I couldn't stand the whispers at school. I was already a freak to most of my classmates. I couldn't also be deemed a sucker.

After I broke up with Mike and stopped spending weekends at his house, my parents never asked me what happened. In keeping with the silence about my first relationship, there wasn't one "Where's Mike?" or "Are you okay?" or "Are you going out?" uttered. They could not acknowledge that I had broken up with my boyfriend if they refused to acknowledge that I was anything other than a gymnast.

Miserable as I was, I didn't seriously entertain the idea of quitting gymnastics. After all my family had sacrificed and my coaches had invested, it was out of bounds. But Mike provided a needed escape during my senior year. He let me cry and dream of life without the sport. He watched me eat ice cream, and it made him smile that I enjoyed it so much. He was just what I needed, someone outside of my very limited world, a drunken high school boy with a surprising perspective. Until I met Mike, I had been driving without headlights. Suddenly, I was aware of the entire highway, not very well lit, but leading anywhere I chose to take it.

After the breakup, I had no support in my immediate world and my depression deepened. Every moment felt backward, elongated and reversed, pulling me further away from my future. All I thought about was finishing high school, getting through another year of training, and putting gymnastics behind me. And with every passing minute it seemed further and further away. Time inverted, youth and freedom seemed desperately unreachable. And as my melancholy escalated, so did the conflict at home. Despair about my situation, the perceived lack of choice, opened up an ugly anger in me and created a great divide in my family. I fought with my mother, feuds that created a chasm for years to come.

When I caught my mom rifling through my secret laxative stash, I chose not to announce myself. I watched her from the doorway to my room as she refolded my clothes, neatly placing them back on top of the boxes of pills. I hoped that she would confront me, having discovered the most obvious sign of my self-inflicted abuse and desperate emotional state. She must have shared her discovery with my father, a doctor's advice the obvious next step. She might have suggested that he discuss it with me. My father and I didn't fight; his commitment to my gymnastics was less rigorous than my mom's, and his resentment toward my waning devotion was less ardent. But neither of them ever mentioned it. No one intervened. To this day, my mom and I have never spoken of this incident specifically or my laxative abuse in general.

When Mrs. Strauss threw me out of the gym until I lost three pounds, the fighting with my mother intensified. The subsequent week without practice allowed me to get a glimpse of a life without the sport. Barely a peek and the fog lifted, ever so slightly. It wasn't bad, I thought. No daily fear and pain and humiliation. I considered leaving for college upon graduation, rather than waiting the extra year to train for the Olympics. It wouldn't be quitting, I reasoned. Just moving on with life. I'd applied and been accepted to Stanford University. Rather than defer as planned, I told my mom I wanted to enter in 1987, class of 1991. To stop competing now, while I was ahead. She was furious.

"No! You won't!" she screamed.

I was dumbstruck. "It's my choice!" I raged. I believed that it was indeed my choice, that I could choose to quit and live with the potential regret.

She struck back. "No it isn't! You'll regret it. I won't let it happen! You're going back to the gym on Monday!" Though I was nearly eighteen years old, my mom acted as if I was a child of ten and she wielded total control over my decisions. In many ways I was mature beyond my years, but I was dependent and, to date, unrebellious. This lack of manifest revolt had delayed my transition to adulthood in my mother's eyes.

Now was my time to rebel. I told her I wouldn't lose the weight and they wouldn't take me back in the gym. This was my first act of real independence. I used my body to assert control over my life. And, inverting the anorexic paradigm of maintaining control and little-girl status by starving, I proclaimed my adulthood by gaining weight. My mom lost control, threatening imposed starvation. "I won't let you eat! I'll lock the cabinets! You're not going to throw this away after all the time and money we've spent! Not after moving to this godforsaken town!"

I grabbed her, shook her with every angry fiber, every sad moment. I wanted to hit her, wanted it more than anything. I knew I was stronger, that I could hurt her, but I just couldn't do it. I released her and fled to my room as she slumped to the floor.

It would have taken so little for my mom or my dad to diffuse the situation. To reach me would have been so easy. A simple "It's going to be okay. Whatever happens, it will be okay" might have even given me the impetus to proceed. If my mom had reached out to me, grabbed my hand, told me she knew how hard it was; if she had recognized that I was harming myself, offered to help me get better; if my dad had hugged me and told me I could be whatever I wanted, as he had done in the ambulance in Montreal—any such small but honest gesture of concern and empathy would have been all that I needed. To continue or not. But all that I needed to find the resolve to go forward. Whichever path I chose.

But my mom had dedicated every waking moment to my young career. And my dad was complicit. He had let her forsake their marriage in giving herself over to my gymnastics. His silent acquiescence provided approval, and he couldn't go back now. Her mistake was his as well. Their transition from supportive and proud mom and dad to emotionally neglectful stage parents was quiet and seamless. And, ultimately, understandable, given all that they'd sacrificed. But at this point, for either of them to reach beyond my mom's calamitous disappointment would be admitting failure.

A year of fighting culminated in yet another U.S. Championships, which I almost chose not to attend. The months leading up to the competition were tumultuous. I could barely perform the simplest moves anymore. I was completely undone. One afternoon, the gym was relatively empty, with all of the other girls out at nationals. I had already secured my spot at championships, placing third in the first qualifier of the season. Even in my unhinged state, I'd been able to pull out an acceptable performance. A seasoned competitor, I made routines in the meet that I rarely hit in practice.

Since then, things had worsened. Audrey Schweyer, a judge who consulted for our team, had shown her disgust a week earlier during a visit to our gym. I was practicing balance beam, preparing for the second national meet. She shook her head in dismay as I dismounted the beam after falling twice during the routine.

"You really shouldn't wear your hair that way anymore," she said. "It makes your face look fat." She pushed my bangs off of my forehead. "And you know, doing gymnastics at your weight is like doing it with a ten-pound bag of sugar strapped to your back." She paused to let her words sink in, then gave me a pat on the shoulder. "Why don't you try again."

I hopped back up onto the beam for another go as she tsked-tsked with Mrs. Strauss. I fell again. She recommended to Mrs. Strauss that I not attend the upcoming nationals. It would be embarrassing for both the team and for me, she reasoned. And it wasn't necessary. Perhaps I could get it together before championships if I stayed at home and trained. Mrs. Strauss agreed. So I stayed in Allentown while the other Parkettes went off to compete. A few months later when I read in *The Morning Call* that Mrs. Schweyer had been arrested at a local department store for shoplifting a cheap costume necklace, I felt vindicated.

Having stayed at home as instructed, I engaged in a one-on-one session in a very quiet gym with a new coach, Fico. His patience enabled me to relearn some of my bar moves. I started the day "ripping off"—unable to hold on midrotation around the bar, my body was flung from the pole, leaving it twanging as I flew across the mat, landing on my head, my back, my stomach. Repeatedly. Finally, after countless attempts, I was able to hold on and complete the skill, a Stalder full (a 360-degree rotation around the bar, legs in the straddled position, culminating in a full pirouette on the hands). I was lighthearted for the first time in a year, grateful for his understanding. Fico had been a gymnast, and he knew sometimes things didn't come easily. He understood how tricks could be unlearned, then relearned.

While Fico and I were joking by the chalk dish in between turns, Mrs. Strauss crashed in like a tornado. She came back early from the meet to ensure that I was making appropriate progress before championships. Fico suggested I show off my remastered Stalder pirouette. My elevated mood and modest improvements were not enough for Mrs. Strauss, who expected transformation. She demanded a contender at the upcoming USA's. She wanted to see a whole routine, a near-10.0 performance. She exploded with epithets and anger.

"This is it! You think this is good enough? I leave you here for a week, and all you have to show me is something you could do a year ago? Where's the rest of it?"

I sat, head bowed, as Fico defended me. "She just got it back. First things first. Patience," he urged.

"You're not even trying! You're the national champion, and you're going to go to championships like *that*? Jesus! And you're fat. What did you weigh today?" She was inconsolable. Unreasonable.

I couldn't take it anymore. I stood up for myself for the first time, no longer afraid of this fiery, demanding woman. When she accused me of not trying, of being lazy, I lost it. After years of punishing hard work, painful injury, and emotional abuse, how dare she accuse me of laziness? I grabbed my gym bag, slipped on my sneakers, and left. I didn't say a word. I walked all the way home, three miles, through sketchy downtown Allentown, wearing nothing but a leotard and sneakers.

I figured, I hoped, I'd be expelled for good. But sure enough, knowing that they couldn't suffer the embarrassment of not having their former champ show up at this year's competition to defend her title, Mr. Strauss called and apologized for his wife. He begged me to come back to the gym. I complied.

Upon reentry, I decided upon a new approach. I'd try anything they asked of me with the hope that I'd injure myself. I would recklessly embark upon the most difficult skills, moves I would generally be wary of attempting. Without a second thought, I would throw my body around. Without visualization, without hesitation. The crowning devastating trauma would be my own doing. I would instigate my own demise, embarking on the career-ending injury with total intent.

Unfortunately, or fortunately, it had the opposite effect. I was pulled from the depths of incompetence; recklessness restored my abilities. I learned new tricks, world-class skills. I performed multiple release moves in my bar routine, twisting and spinning on the event that had always given me such trouble. I landed full twisting double backs on floor and double pike dismounts off the balance beam. I was flying again, though the joy of it was gone. I was indifferent to each new skill I mastered, and I continued to pray for injury.

Two weeks before 1987 U.S. Championships, despite my recent surge of ability, I decided I was finished. Regardless of physical improvement, the fact remained that I was miserable. Distraught, I took half a box of laxatives one Sunday morning. I wanted to incapacitate myself, cause such weakness that I'd have to take to my bed come Monday. By that evening I was volcanic. I couldn't even make it to the toilet. My mom had invited a new girl at the gym, along with her mother, over for dinner. She was welcoming them to our home as I scrambled toward the bathroom, leaking a humiliating trail of diarrhea behind me. I was reduced to shitting in my pants in front of an innocent and still-hopeful gymnast. I had lost all dignity. Feigning illness, I retreated to my bedroom and sobbed. All I wanted was for all of this to end—the treacherous practices, the gut-wrenching competitions, the starvation and self-flagellation. I simply knew I could not continue. Even monthly cortisone shots did nothing to alleviate the pain and swelling in my ankle. But I was afraid. I knew no life without gymnastics. I didn't know myself without it.

When I told my mother that I would not attend the upcoming championships, that I was going to call it quits, she threatened back. She said she wouldn't attend my high school graduation. She would, in essence, disavow our relationship. Complete and total rejection. She told me I was a failure. That nothing I'd accomplished amounted to anything if I didn't stick it out until 1988. I cried and gasped for air between sobs. When she shrieked "Failure!" I grabbed her and dug my fingers into her arms. As I pushed her against the wall, I wanted to slam her head into it. Her betrayal felt so merciless. I wanted to hurt her as she hurt me, but I released her, barely containing myself.

With coaxing from my father, my mom relented and attended my graduation. And I conceded and attended the meet. I went into it with the most careless attitude I could muster. Michelle Dusserre, a 1984 Olympian and fellow veteran, another girl who'd struggled with injuries and comebacks, was in my rotation group. We made a pact: we were going to enjoy this competition. For the first time, we were going to have fun. Ignore the jitters, the pressure, and bask in the pride of being a part of it all. And we did. I'd never had so much fun in a meet. I surprised everyone, my coaches most of all, who assumed I'd have a disastrous competition despite insisting I attend. I'd barely practiced at all in the weeks leading up to it. I was told by Mrs. Schweyer that I'd embarrass myself looking like I did. She repeatedly emphasized my ten-pound handicap, comparing it to a ten-pound bag of potatoes.

On my first event during optionals day, I hurled my body down the vaulting runway to perform a Yurchenko, the latest skill, the apex of difficulty. Named for Natalia Yurchenko, a former Soviet World Champion Team medalist, the vault featured a round-off onto the board and a back handspring onto the horse. This approach provided more power than I'd ever been able to summon. I performed it with a layout full twist off the horse to the floor, garnering a 9.9. I was overjoyed. One fall on bars allowed me a seventh all-around placement, officially qualifying me for the World Championship Team for the second time.

Kristie Phillips, the junior champ from the prior year, won the meet as expected. She was celebrated as the United States' hope for the upcoming Olympics. Before her win as a senior, she had already landed herself the cover of *Sports Illustrated,* the youngest cover athlete ever featured, touted as "the next Mary Lou." Her glory and fame proved temporary. In 1988, just one year later, she would suffer her own devastating disappointment by missing the Olympic Team, despite the excitement and frenzied publicity over her potential. And after this very public demise, she would attempt a comeback at the age of twenty-seven, more than ten years later. I interpreted this failed comeback as an inability to find her place in the world beyond gymnastics. An inability to reconcile her successes and failures. A need to rectify the failures, no matter what the cost. It was a pitiable circumstance. I watched her return to the sport with empathy and sadness. At the 1999 U.S. Championships, Kristie placed twenty-third in the all-around, proving that gymnastics is indeed a young girl's sport. She would have to make peace with both her accomplishments and failures after all.

I was satisfied with my performance in championships, the sixth such meet of my career. I felt proud even though I had slid six places since 1986; even though my nemesis from the prior year triumphed, proving all the judges and coaches right that she was the better gymnast. Many champions failed to even make the team the year after their victory. Sabrina Mar, the 1985 champ, didn't make the top ten in her follow-up year. Kristie, so vaunted at this year's meet, would place ninth in the subsequent year. Sustained performance and ranking were elusive, so I was satisfied with making the world team, no matter how far I'd fallen. The effort it had taken to get here, to endure the year of training, made this meet a true victory. And once again, I toyed with the idea of walking away.

# Chapter 26

I'd earned a spot on both the Pan American and World Championship Teams. I had assumed that the meet was going to be such a disaster that there would be no need to continue training, my failure writ large upon the wall. As this had not been the case, quitting remained illusive. My hanging on to a U.S. team spot seduced me into believing that staying in the sport for one more year might not be so bad. The Strausses and John had gotten me this far. I was already miserable. What was another year? I deferred my admission to Stanford, agreeing to enter with the high school class of 1988. And now that I wasn't quitting, I was immediately faced with another hurdle: the Pan Am Games.

I attended the training camp and was berated for my weight, despite the fact that I had whittled it down to 102 pounds. At eighteen years of age and almost five feet four, I considered this acceptable. The nutritionist disagreed. She called me to her office, sat me down with a stern glare. She asked if there were struggles with weight in the family.

"Is your mom overweight?"

"No."

"Your dad?"

I shook my head.

"Siblings?" she pressed.

"A brother. He's not fat either," I mumbled.

"Then what's wrong with you?" I was humiliated. My body-fat test had come back at 3 percent, higher than some of the younger girls, yes. But high? I was officially a young woman, two years shy of my twentieth birthday, and I still had never gotten my period. She suggested a "diet" rich in vegetables and whole grains and about four times the calories I normally ate in a day. I left the training camp early on my own volition.

Ironically, demonstrating the capacity for independent decision making landed me in the "past her prime" category. I was officially over the hill. Self-determined behavior was considered a detriment to championship performance. While I considered leaving Parkettes to try to jump-start my career, get back some of the motivation, no other team wanted me at this point.

I spiraled downward. My previous approach of throwing anything and everything, hoping to sustain injury, was no longer working. I couldn't summon the strength. I could barely get out of bed each day, let alone throw my body through the air. I took to skipping practices, something I'd never done before. I'd drive to the mall, wandering the food court or just sitting in the parking lot, crying. After a few hours, figuring my mother was sufficiently worried, I'd drive home. Distraught that I hadn't been training (the coaches called looking for me), she was locked away in her room.

Dr. Dixon finally diagnosed my foot. After nearly two years

of pain, he found multiple bone chips, floating around in the ankle. He said they had taken years to calcify, preventing detection on earlier X-rays. Tiny chips, floating aimlessly, causing trouble. Some became lodged in the joint, causing irritation and infection, one time leading to a high fever. Dr. Dixon said that I could have them removed, but that I would be out of the gym for a while. The coaches said no. I had survived with them for this long; why take them out now? Surgery could wait until retirement. Until Stanford.

After storming out of Pan Am training camp, I refused to go to World Championships. I was a stumbling, limping, blathering, sobbing mess. The Strausses were relieved, though they wouldn't admit it. I would have embarrassed them if I had gone to that training camp. I was an alternate going in with my seventh-place ranking, and undoubtedly, my performance would not have convinced anyone of my worthiness to compete.

Somewhere in my foggy mental state, I finally found the strength to confront my mother. I had stumbled on a solution I thought she could accept. I would continue training. But not at Parkettes. I would go back to Lolo's, the only club that would have me. She'd provide the nurturing environment that I needed. In a moment of clarity, I knew that if I could get away from my mother, the Strausses, even John, who still believed I'd recover from all of this, Lolo would help me find my way back to mental health. At this point, my parents bickered constantly over my future in the sport. My dad had come around to letting me disappear from gymnastics. It wasn't worth it to him anymore. He allowed that I could take my winnings and escape to college, putting the whole affair behind me. Us. My mother fought him bitterly over this concession. But eventually he convinced her to let me go back to Will-Moor.

The Parkette coaches were furious. Robin took it upon herself to confront me. Since I had graduated from high school and was no longer busy with classes during the day, I had taken a retail job stocking and folding to fill the morning hours. Robin accosted me in the parking lot of the discount clothier the day after I tendered my resignation to the Strausses.

"Don't do this," she pleaded. "Just quit. You can't leave and go somewhere else. Do you know how this looks for us? A former national champion, going to another gym?"

I wanted to scream, "It's not your choice! It's my choice! And I *want* to quit, but my mother won't let me!"

Listening to her made me want to give it an honest try at Lolo's, if only out of spite.

I packed my things and headed back to New Jersey. My family stayed in Allentown, a cruel and bitter irony. My dad commuted to Philadelphia each day and my brother continued to train at Gymnastrum. Chris was a junior at Allen High, and he wanted to graduate with his friends. For once, he got his way. All of the girls who had lived with us had moved on already. Jen went to UCLA and Kristy went to Berkeley. Alyssa was a year younger than us and had gone home to New Jersey for a year before starting college; she would be joining me at Stanford. Ultimately, everyone fled the grayness of Allentown for sunny California. My mom was left with my brother and the occasional temporary gymnastics boarder. I left them all there, mired in gymnastics and resentment, probably glad, at least a little bit, to be free of me. I moved in with my aunt Jill, who had been ever-present and always supportive throughout my career. And I slacked.

I knew that I'd chosen to return to Lolo to find love and understanding. To rehabilitate myself. She had always appreciated me as a person, not a gymnast. Being an athlete had been incidental and temporary in her mind. A few years earlier this had frustrated me; now I craved this kind of acceptance. If I found my way back to gymnastics with her, fine. But it wasn't the goal. Becoming an adult was.

Lolo's was a safe haven where I could ease into retirement without anyone noticing. And again, for the second time, she welcomed me with open arms. She didn't care if I didn't show up for practice. She didn't care if I showed up and didn't do anything but stretch and chat with the other girls. She gave me classes to teach. She hugged me often. Her son Sam, formerly fat, was now a weight lifter and trained me on free weights. I bench-pressed, curled, and squatted. I built bulky muscle. He shaped my physical strength, a proxy and precursor for emotional wherewithal.

Lolo reminded me that I was the 1986 national champion, a claim no one else could make. She made it clear that I had a whole life stretched before me.

A life without gymnastics. A life that included friends and family, college and career, marriage and kids, whatever I chose. These were things I'd never considered, caught in the desperate dark tunnel of gymnastics.

My depression took a year to diminish in its intensity. My laxative use worsened now that I was free to buy them whenever I wanted. I had a car and no one hovering over my shoulder. I bought boxes at a time at the pharmacy, buried beneath other manufactured list items like Band-Aids and baby powder. I often thought of crashing my car, veering across the median, as I drove the highway on the way to practice. Distraught and hopeless about my family situation, I no longer spoke with my parents at all. Their disappointment in me was unabated. Mine in them was intensified. No more screaming, just silence. If I thought about my mother, I couldn't breathe.

While living with Jill, I received a beseeching letter from my father. He came short of an apology and urged me to consider my mother's circumstances, to take pity on her and come home before college. She had my best interest at heart, he insisted. She wanted to protect me from disappointment later in life. She was out of line, yes. But for the right reasons, he claimed. The letter was printed, bit-map style; his word processor was his latest toy. I was incensed. In the days before the ubiquity of computers, the fact that he didn't handwrite the letter felt impersonal, bordering on vulgar. And I was intent on finding any reason not to go back home. I was going to make them work to repair the damage they'd done. I tore up the letter, scrawled a handwritten note in response: "You're more enamored of experimenting with your new computer than you are in me. Where's the apology? Where's *Mom's* letter?"

I attended one competition with Lolo. It was horrendous. Devastatingly embarrassing. Tucked away at an unimportant meet in the unassuming state of Alabama, I fell on every event, usually more than once. Not only did I fall, I tripped and stumbled, appeared a clumsy fool. After the meet, I sobbed tears of humiliation. I choked and gasped as I pondered the depths of my disgrace. It was inconceivable that this could all end in such ruination and indignity. I cried the tears of an ending. I cried because I feared that all I'd accomplished had been the Strausses' doing. That I was nothing without them. That I had no present in the sport and no future without it. And I cried for weeks after, when I returned to New Jersey. The choking tears gave way to weeping. I pedaled the exercise bike while Sam listened and tears streamed down my face.

And then one day I stopped crying. The tears had cleansed and made way for the undeniable truth: I was done. There would be no Olympic Trials or 1988 Olympics in my future. There would be no crowning accomplishment that would wash away the pain and repair the vast and ugly rift in my family. My greatest achievement in the sport was behind me. I would bide my time until I could leave for college, out to California, far away from my mother's disapproving glare and never-ending disappointment. And I would start anew.

I arrived at Stanford on crutches. I'd finally had the nagging bone chips removed from my ankle, though a few remain to this day. I hobbled around campus, struck by the energy and accomplishment of my fellow freshmen. Many of the kids there were also athletes. They played tennis and football and basketball. Most envisioned a career well beyond college, in the pros. Some would achieve it, making their life a life of sport, gleaning a lifetime of satisfaction from their superior athletic ability, their mastery of a game. Alex O'Brien, a freshman dorm mate, would become a U.S. Open tennis champ in doubles, achieving the number-one ranking in the world. Dave McCarty, another dorm resident, would play professional baseball for a host of teams including the Kansas City Royals and the Boston Red Sox. Ed McCaffrey, a fellow Allentownian, would become a wide receiver for the Denver Broncos, winning three Super Bowl rings during the course of his career. I envied these athletes. Their childhood prowess became their adult identity. Whether they were athletes or not, all the kids approached college with the gusto of birth. They kicked and screamed, energized by their new surroundings. Out on their own for the first time, they were giddy with possibility.

I was enervated, completely exhausted. I viewed college as a retirement home, a place where I could finally rest. I didn't think there was life beyond these four years right in front of me. This was the end for me. For so long, I'd strived to get here so that I could simply rest. For so long, I'd wanted nothing more than to not be a gymnast anymore. And now that I had these things, I didn't know who I was. I was lost.

And so I ate. I ate to become another person. Someone I might know. I gained forty pounds my freshman year, transforming myself from a lean world-class athlete into a puffy round ball. Early during my freshman year, amidst the frenzy of this massive weight pile-on, I started menstruating. At age twenty, I had no idea how to use a tampon. Alyssa, my former Parkette teammate, housemate, and now fellow co-ed, showed me how. I struggled, unsure where these womanly body parts she was describing were located. We laughed while Alyssa ushered me into womanhood in a way my mother could not.

Four hazy years of eating, drinking, and forgetting, and it finally dawned on me. I hadn't even started yet. I was barely twenty-three years old, mature for a senior due to my deferment. But, with graduation imminent, I finally understood that I had to carve a life for myself beyond gymnastics. I had to start my life, for real this time, without the concocted pressures of gymnastics, the conjured, artificial meaning of competition.

Today, at thirty-eight, I've discovered my life, but my body haunts me. I'm all too aware of its earthly weightiness. With each step across the pavement, my beaten ankles shock. The balls of my feet, permanently bruised from gymnastics, ache with every stride. My knees grind and creak each time I rise from a chair. My back shoots sciatic reminders down my legs at a family outing to the park. I pretend not to notice. My hands are swollen and stiff each morning when I wake; because of arthritis and a disorder called "trigger finger" (which generally only afflicts aging diabetic men) it takes an hour for the fluid to drain enough that I can wear my wedding ring or comfortably hold a cup of coffee. Every movement reminds me that I'm mortal.

Yet, every day, I miss the feeling of flying. I will never

experience it again. Sometimes, if I run far enough, past my limits, I can beat my legs into numbness, almost replicating the feeling of being a young gymnast on a good day. I can make myself feel numb but heavy. Never light. And I always feel the pain later. I pay the price with sore shins, aching ankles, and "hip pointers" jabbing into my pelvis.

Still, I have a love affair with gymnastics, with that period in my life. Often, I dream dreams of weightlessness. When I feel most disheartened, heavy with the burdens of everyday life, I imagine myself buoyant, floatable. I waft, on my own accord, propelled by my own volition, in effortless control. Completely powerful, resilient, substantial, agile.

I miss it every day.

2000

FEELINGS OF FAILURE FOLLOW ME. NOT FAILURE ITSELF, BUT
the feeling of never being good enough. I am thirty-one
years old, and I am just home from the hospital, having had
my first child. I am dead set on breast-feeding him because
that is what the best and most caring mothers do. I am not
sure I will be able to, though. When I was in my twenties, after years of abusing my body, eating and eating and gaining
and gaining, my weight ballooned and so did my breasts. I had
surgery to cut them down to a reasonable size, to hide the
shame of my out-of-control appetite.

I am at home with my husband when my milk comes in.
It's one in the morning, and Virgil, my three-day-old son, is
screaming because he's hungry. My breasts are hard and lumpy.
I am heartened, as the doctors weren't sure that I would lac-
tate. Now the test. Will I be able to feed him? The doctors
can't tell me whether the ducts that carry milk from my

breasts to my son are functional. I will just have to try it, they tell me.

I get him into position. We've been practicing "latching on" for the past few days. Even though nothing but goopy yellow stuff has been emitted, he sucks like a demon. This bodes well, I think. Now that there is milk, he will be happy. He quiets for a bit. He gulps heartily and I am relieved. And then, just minutes into this process, he pulls away, arching his back and squealing. He kicks and cries and I am desperate to get him to stop, to bring him some comfort. Maybe that was it? Maybe there isn't any more milk? I squeeze the nipple and nothing comes out. I am steeped in shame. My body doesn't work the way a mother's body is supposed to work. I cannot feed my son adequately. He will suffer because of me and my failures and my boundless shame.

And now I feel shame on top of shame because, once disgraced as a gymnast, I could not accept my post-gymnastics body. I couldn't leave well enough alone. I had to slice myself up into pieces to give the appearance of being in control. The repercussions of this sport are endless. They reach beyond any assumptions I could have made. They go beyond tenuous body image and regret over not having stuck it out until the bitter end. The shame is never-ending. I didn't win the time I was supposed to. I didn't stay divinely thin, above the normal everyday fray of human need and hunger. I am not better than I am.

I find myself today, twelve years after my last day in the gym, having to overcome the same profound sense of inadequacy that I felt when I was nineteen. Did I learn nothing? Why have I not yet learned to accept the present state of things, to pivot toward the future so that new good things can come my way? Maybe not better than the ones in the past or the ones I'd hoped for. But good things nonetheless. It is a lesson I will have to learn over and over again. It is one I will never remember when faced with a future different from the one I planned for myself.

In a heap on the bathroom floor, wrestling with my infant, trying again and again to get him to eat, I feel a colossal sense of failure. It is now three-thirty in the morning, and I rock him and apologize for my weakness as I fill a bottle with formula. This bottle will become a symbol of my shame that will send ripples of humiliation to my face and head and heart every time I have to give him one. I will nurse him persistently, hoping it will change things, that I will restore my body to its intended form. But I will always have to fill in with bottles. To supplement my love with manufactured powdered milk brings terrible and deep feelings of botched competence and self-hatred.

I will have to learn to forgive myself. I will have to move on, past this one aspect of mothering. I will have to be better at the other parts, to make up for this failure.

# Afterword

I WAS COMPELLED TO WRITE THIS story, despite the self-indulgence of it all, because the dreams of gymnastics still plague me. There are worse things, and I know this, than being stalked by memories of championship-level performance. They color every day, every decision, every thought about myself. Having been the best at something at a very young age, it is inevitable that anything less than number-one status provokes feelings of failure. *I have been in my job without a promotion for three years. I'm a failure. I work too much and I am not at home enough with my children. I'm a failure. My son isn't the smartest in his class. I'm a failure. My youngest doesn't talk. He's three and not talking. I'm a failure. My husband and I fight. I'm a failure. We don't have enough money. We can't do all the stupid things that I don't even want to do like go on vacation to Mexico or Hawaii and buy a vacation home in Napa Valley. Or even a regular home in San Francisco. I'm a failure.* As a professional, a mother, a wife. How can I ever be the best at anything ever again? And even if I was the best at any of these things, how would I know? My winning days are long behind me. Everything since is proof of my not-up-to-snuff-ness.

In addition to the dreams, there are issues with my mother that persist. Not so unlike issues any daughter has with her mother but somehow in my mind, inextricably related to my gymnastics days. Especially the insecurity she has about our relationship. Twenty years after our battles, she feels unsure that I will forgive her. She carries a mother's self-reproach, certain that every time her child suffers, she could have been the one to prevent it. She believes I live three thousand miles away from her because I cannot stand to live closer. She can't conceive that I simply prefer California to Philadelphia.

When I was giving birth to my first child and chose to have a doctor friend (Doe, from my competition days) present along with my husband instead of my mother, she took this as a sign that I didn't want her in my life. To her, this was incontrovertible proof that I would never forgive her for the missteps of my rearing. It took days of tearful conversations to convince her otherwise. It was her inability to keep a cool head under pressure that caused me to banish her from the labor room, not the fact that she gave up her life so that I could do gymnastics and then lost her mind when I didn't want to do it anymore. Asking her to wait outside the delivery room was not my way of asking her to stay out of my life.

Besides the bad dreams and the flawed but reasonably close relationship with my mom, the result of my gymnastics experience is that I am a bit of an overachiever. Or more likely, that is just what I am and gymnastics was its first manifestation. If my friends—some of whom have known me since my days as a gymnast—were asked to describe me, I think that they would say I am well adjusted and confident. A dedicated mother, friend, sister, wife, daughter. I am a part of all these things. But I am also anxious, sad, self-loathing, impatient, angry, frustrated, competitive, bordering on unhinged at times. And always in constant motion, maniacally desperate for salvation. I am the same now as I was then.

I work myself to the brink of exhaustion to suppress the feelings of being not good enough. I have worked in marketing for nearly fifteen years, and many would be envious of my position as a junior-level executive. I am consistently lauded at my company and within the industry, yet I maintain a coach/athlete relationship with my superiors, always striving for approval, never feeling good enough. Berating myself for every misstep, before it's been called out. Sure that someone better is just around the corner and that my "coach" will choose her to take my place. I carry this self-eradicating, desperate need for recognition with me in everything that I do.

Despite professional achievement, this career has always been a fallback for me. I always thought I would do something special, less average. But fearing the repercussions of *less average* (that hadn't gone so well the first time), I took my first *real* job at an advertising agency when I was twenty-four.

I'd been biding my time in San Francisco after graduating from college. The city was in the throes of a recession hangover, and high unemployment rates meant difficulty securing a first job. Though I'd been offered one in New York as the assistant to a film producer (the father of my gym friend and former housemate Jen), I didn't want to be on the East Coast. California had seduced me with its temperate climate, beautiful architecture, and open-mindedness. Feisty and intent on making it on my own, I took a job teaching gymnastics to unpromising and undedicated girls at a low-level club outside of San Francisco. It was a desperate move, but I made nearly twenty dollars an hour, versus the minimum wage my college friends were bringing in working retail or waiting tables. While I coached in a musty gym, reminiscent of every gym I ever trained or competed in, I often felt impatient and riled, and I raised my voice with these young girls. I resented having to coach. I recognized that my lack of equanimity meant I should not continue, not that I had ever intended to in the long run.

I doubled my efforts in the job search and was offered a position at a well-regarded advertising agency in San Francisco. I told myself it would just be for a little while, until I figured out what I wanted. But I had a knack for it. I liked the respect I garnered. It satisfied my need for recognition. The rapid promotions benefited my self-esteem, boundless in its hunger. Still, I felt average. So what if I became the best account manager in one agency in one city? Didn't that put me amidst the masses?

I quit a few jobs, emboldened with the learning from my late gymnastics experience—I could remove myself from unpleasantness. Any unpleasantness at all, no matter how insignificant. If I didn't like my boss, I could leave and find a more amenable situation. But I always went back to marketing, rife with anxiety as the need for consistent income and positive feedback outweighed the need to explore my true but unrevealed passions. The thought of writing lurked, but I was too afraid to start something new. I wouldn't be any good. My "creative" friends had been writing throughout college; they went on to get their graduate degrees while I got promoted to senior marketing manager. It was too late to start now, I reasoned.

I met my husband, Winslow Warren, while I was working at the advertising agency. He was cautious and kind, funny in an unexpected way. When we met at a party, he asked me what I did for a living.

"How would you advertise black men to white women?" he asked. He was a black man, asking a white woman; this was a funny question. Oddly flirtatious. Clever.

"What's the unique selling proposition?" I winced as the words passed my lips, knowing where this was going.

"Well, I don't want to say. It would be bragging." We laughed as he continued the line of suggestive questioning. He was an environmental chemist. At six feet eight inches tall, under two hundred pounds, he was skinny, chronically mournful, and self-deprecating. Right up my alley. Our courtship was easy and relatively uneventful. He didn't play games. He showed up at my house unannounced, called me every day, and told me that I was beautiful even though I thought I was obese. At times he became disconsolate and withdrawn. His despair did not dissuade me; it drew me closer. After a year, we moved in together.

Winslow learned early on about my history in gymnastics. It came up often.

"I dated a girl from Stanford who was your year. But she was younger than you. Were you held back?" He smirked when he said this.

"I waited a year to go to college."

"Why?"

"It's a long story."

In 1996 we watched the Olympics together. When Kerri Strug collapsed after her first vault and proceeded to perform a second, she helped the American team secure a gold medal. While Winslow was impressed with her tenacity, I was angered by the commentators calling her out as unique. "Any girl on that team would have done the same thing. Why didn't anyone question the fact that she did it? Maybe she shouldn't have competed with a broken ankle!" He learned his lesson.

And in 1998, when he was watching U.S. Championships

on television while I urged him to change the channel from my post at the stove, the announcer celebrated Kristen Maloney's triumph as "the first Parkette win since 1986, when Jennifer Sey took the title!" Winslow was flabbergasted. "They said your name!" He was finally fully convinced I hadn't made the whole thing up.

Though my childhood was markedly different from his (him: black, midwestern non-Jew), our dedication to hard work matched with our ambivalence about corporate work life bonded us. We were reluctant professionals, dedicated Generation Xers. We prided ourselves in our malcontentedness. We knew better than to be happy when we would just end up disappointed, so we distracted ourselves with counterculture parties. The rave era in San Francisco was in full swing, and we often enjoyed all-night clubbing replete with designer drugs as well as the more old-fashioned variety. Through the parties and altered states, Winslow and I stayed in love; we never lost our heads. We each maintained our career trajectories, despite our continued seditious dissatisfaction, no longer in vogue during the tech boom in the Bay Area.

On my thirtieth birthday, our wild partying days receding, Winslow proposed. My parents—unwilling to comment positively or negatively on any choice I might make, afraid of causing another decadelong rift—celebrated and threw us a wedding. We got married in Philadelphia on September 12, 2000. Doe, my rival from 1986 championships, was a bridesmaid. She had attended Stanford also and we became close, bonded in our disdain for coaches and the sport of gymnastics. Still rankled by the events of our teen years, things others didn't even know about us, we found solace in each other. Jen, the former skinny Parkette and Sey house boarder, was also in my wedding party. We'd remained friends through the years, our childhood experience bridging the gaps in our adult lives.

My mother planned the entire wedding, my father walked me down the aisle, and my brother was my man of honor. Chris and I had built a solid, trusting friendship while attending college together. He'd gone to Stanford as well, the lure of California, strong academics, and a gymnastics scholarship too great to pass up, even if he had to follow in my footsteps once again. He came to understand the way I suffered at the end of my gymnastics career. I came to appreciate what it must have been like to live in the background of our family. He was, and is, my best friend. At my wedding, after more than a decade of friction, we resembled a well-adjusted family again.

I became pregnant three months after Winslow and I got married. Though I felt unprepared and unsure, I knew that motherhood might be the one thing that could set me straight. I had long ago given up my bulimic behaviors, but I clung to insecurities about my body. When I was stressed, I obsessed, counting calories and exercising compulsively. At my yearly doctor visits, I didn't look at the number on the scale because then, inevitably, I would have to compare it to what I weighed during gymnastics. Winslow was all too aware of my preoccupations. Though I didn't want to broadcast my insecurities as an adult (I refrained from the "Do I look fat?" type of questions), I withdrew when I felt unwieldy. Retreat to the simple to solve weight issues was my go-to when things got tough. Winslow knew this about me and patiently coaxed me away from these behaviors. He didn't do it with cloying sensitivity and hippie-style understanding. He used humor. "Back that up over here. Yeah, it's round! I like it! I'm black!" he'd say in mock ebonics, making me laugh while giving me the acceptance I needed.

Being pregnant, I fought the urge to hate myself. I forced myself to contend with the rising number on the scale, topping 150 only midway through gestation. I came to recognize that my body had a higher purpose, all the while resenting what that purpose did to me.

On September 30, 2000, forty pounds and nine months later, Virgil Warren was born. He taught me that being the best amongst the broadest population is not what matters. It's being loved amidst the narrowest that does. Though I have to remind myself constantly, Virgil is pretty good at helping me to remember. Greeting me with frantic squeals of "Mommy's home!" at the end of a long workday pretty much does the trick.

Wyatt Warren joined Virgil on April 30, 2003. Moody and temperamental, Wyatt reinforces for me that my petty needs and insecurities do not always come first.

But sometimes they do. I will not set myself aside to raise my children. I continue to work, and Winslow stays home with our kids. And some time ago, amidst the nightmares about gymnastics, the nursing of babies, and the exhausting climb up the corporate ladder, I decided that I should try to write.

Fearful of my parents' response, not wanting them to have to relive the guilt that they have wallowed in over the years, I have not shared this book with them. They will have to buy it in the bookstore like average readers. I love them and forgive them, not that forgiveness is required. I could never have achieved the success I did without their blind commitment. They sacrificed themselves and their relationship for a time, to enable my accomplishments. I am a more selfish parent than that. I would never give up my own life to cart Virgil or Wyatt around. While I worry that this may shortchange them in some way, it is the only way I can do this parenting thing. It is a muddy and complicated affair. There is no one telling you what is right or wrong. Each child is different, with different tolerances and needs. Each parent is also unique, with a host of neuroses, dreams, and weaknesses.

As I watched Virgil, age six, at the playground one summer day, it was hard for me not to dissuade him from hanging from his knees on the monkey bars. Big and strong for his age, he is also brave, confident in his physicality. I don't want to be a worrywart. He's a boy, after all. Shouldn't he climb trees, skin knees, break bones? I reminded him to be careful as he called out to me, "Mom, look what I can do!?" I sensed other, more cautious moms, glaring at me, thinking, "He's going to fall and hurt himself. He's going to fall on the other smaller children. How could she?!" These parents of the new millennium, obsessively protecting their kids, are anathema to me. I want my kids to be safe, but I don't want them to live in a bubble. I ignored the other moms, willing to take their angry stares in order to let Virgil sow his oats, find his own limits. I returned my attention to the book I was reading, nervous but forcing myself to let the tether loose.

And then he screamed. I knew his voice without even looking. I ran to him, heaped in a pile on the sand beneath the monkey bars, blood running down his head and neck, staining his shirt. I knew that he was all right—his eyes were focused, his bones intact. But the blood pooled around his left ear and my stomach lurched.

"Virgil bleed, Mommy!" Wyatt screamed.

"I know, baby. I know." My child bled. It was my fault. Just like my mom, I worried that all his pain was my transgression.

I safely tucked Virgil into the car and cleaned him up at home. He whimpered, burying his head in my chest, as I wiped the blood from his neck and tears welled in my eyes.

Wyatt cried in sympathy and fear. Fear of my weepiness more than Virgil's blood. Of course, Virgil was okay, as I'd presumed. A gash on the head, no stitch required. Whew, I thought to myself. Crisis averted.

And then, upon reflection, I thought: My parents were brave. How could they watch me, day after day, throw myself through the most impossible maneuvers, serious injury imminent with each passing moment? How could they watch me crack bones, bleed, cry with pain, without ever insisting that I stop? I used to equate their letting me do gymnastics to letting a child play in traffic. Only a careless parent could watch her daughter run into the street amidst oncoming cars. I took pride in the fact that I would never let my children do gymnastics. I was often asked this question and responded with a dodge: "They'll be too tall." Now, I feel differently.

They will beg to do things that I am not comfortable with. They will do things behind my back that I don't approve of, that I believe may not be in their best interest. I understand that my parents were masters at handling this quandary. They let me swing freely on the monkey bars, putting their own instinctive fears aside to let me feel the joy of becoming who I was meant to be. Disappointment, pain, frustration, and all. This is the greatest challenge for parents. To protect their children while allowing them the room to make real mistakes. Not protected, painless mistakes. But mistakes with true repercussions. Otherwise how will they learn what it is they really want, what wrong turn will cause them to suffer, what is right for them?

As my parents read this, once again, they will watch me become the person I am meant to be. It will pain them some, but they will encourage me. This is what great parents do. They sometimes, not always, set themselves aside, to let their children emerge, become. In doing so, these parents become the best parents. The very best at something that offers no prize other than knowing you've sent a human being into the world who is capable of shining.

I aim to pass the baton, sending Virgil and Wyatt into the world armed and ready to experience disappointment, self-doubt, fear, and joyful exhilaration. I aim to be the best parent, and I strive to fulfill my bestness by not having to measure it at all. I have setbacks all the time. But I've been well prepared to learn from my mistakes.